MORE PRAISE FOR *Becoming Whole:*

"I have read a lot of recovery stories, but none as unflinchingly honest as Meg's. She has totally opened her heart and life and allows the reader to wander around her psyche. This is not only a compelling story, but one of deep truth, open vulnerability and true courage."

Christina Pirello, Author and
Emmy Award Winning Host of Christina Cooks Television Show

"The highest elements of human accomplishments are literally like a religious conversion: a dedication to profoundly correct apocalyptic epiphany. The cover of this book reveals the indomitable human spirit overcoming whatever the obstacle is. Obstacles, in fact, are what you see when you take your eyes off the goal. This book is about taking your eyes off the problem and putting them on the solution. Bravery is demonstrated, health is revealed, perseverance is everything, and all that is herein."

H. Robert Silverstein, MD, F.A.C.C.
Medical Director, Preventive Medicine Center

"This is perhaps the most lurid account I have thus far read of the horrendous treatment journey confronting cancer patients, as well as a positive uplifting, yet authoritative account of a woman's survival from both terminal bone and breast cancer through a Macrobiotic diet. Meg Wolff's book also brings together and summarizes the major scientific and nutritional evidence explaining why a macrobiotic diet may be so effective against cancer."

Sandra Goodman, Ph.D
Editor and Director, Positive Health Publications Ltd

"In *Becoming Whole*, Meg Wolff beautifully and generously invites the reader to become part of her journey to wholeness, offering keen emotional insights every step of the way. This is not just a book for cancer patients, healthy-living enthusiasts, or people struggling with chronic health issues; it is a life-changing gift for all of us."

Julia Mossbridge, author of Unfolding,
The Perpetual Science of Your Soul's Work.

"Meg's story is a real gift to the world. She shows us that wholeness is a verb—not a goal or a fixed state, but a never-ending process of presence and attention, moment by moment, no matter what's happening. She also shows that in real life, integrative medicine is more than just a fruit basket of modalities—it is really a very personal journey of self-awakening. Thank you, Meg!"

William Collinge, Ph.D., author, principal investigator of The COUPLES
Project (NCI study), and consultant in integrative health care

Flow Books
P.O. 213, Cape Elizabeth,
Maine 04104-0213

Set in 11.5 pt on 18 pt Adobe Caslon Pro

cover photograph by Joyce Tenneson
cover and interior design by Carly Schnur

ISBN 13: 978-1-4303-0961-1
ISBN 10: 1-4303-0961-X

NOTE TO THE READER: The macrobiotic lifestyle and health regime described in this book is intended as a vehicle or mechanism by which change can be self-wrought, and in no event should orthodox medical treatment be abandoned. This book is a tool, but only one of many needed, by which profound self-transformation can be achieved.

Becoming Whole

THE STORY OF MY COMPLETE RECOVERY FROM BREAST CANCER

MEG WOLFF

WITH TOM MONTE

DECEMBER 2006

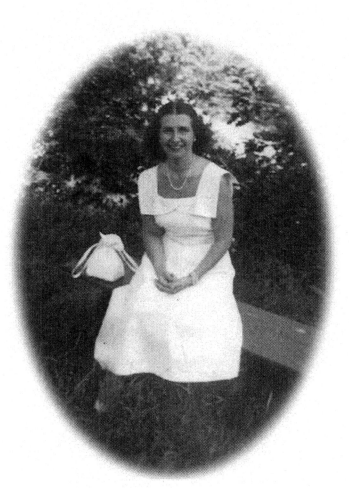

This book is dedicated to my mother, Dolores Bettez DeCoste, my grandmothers, Martha Kane DeCoste and Mary Letarte Bettez, all my female ancestors who came before them, to my daughter, Cammie, my baby—keep being your SELF, and to all the woman that will come after her.

o o o

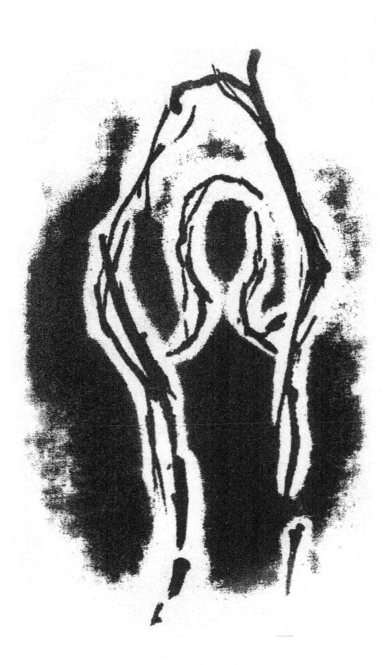

"Although the world is full of suffering, it is also full of overcoming it."

—Helen Keller

"We are each of us angels with only one wing,
and we can only fly by embracing one another."

—*Luciano de Crescenzo*

ACKNOWLEDGMENTS ○ I'd like to acknowledge all the angels in my life. First of all my husband, Tom Wolff, the love of my life who has supported me every step of the way and has challenged me to grow as a person, my children, Francis and Cammie, for having to be different, but not feeling inferior; Eileen Beasley, who believed in me which helped me to believe in my self; Lisa Silverman, Jessica Porter, and Howard Wallen who nourished me with their food and love when I needed it; my sister, Liz Bennett, who makes me laugh out loud and for being my sister; my dad, J. Mark DeCoste, for my open-mindedness and for giving me Jean Kohler's book, *Healing Miracles from Macrobiotics*; my other mom and dad, Charlie and Alice Wolff, who welcomed me into their family wholeheartedly; Tom Monte for writing my story and his wife, Toby, for her support in this project; Aveline and Michio Kushi for bringing health food to America and devoting their lives to helping others; Warren Kramer for sharing his wisdom; Joyce Tenneson a true lightworker, who agreed to do my portrait; Carly Schnur, for her unbridled enthusiasm and cover design; Alex Jack, Luchi Baranda, Carry Wolf, John Kozinski, and Charles Millman—my teachers at the Kushi Institute in Becket, Massachusetts; Mirea Ellis, Olaf Fischer, and Judy and Larry McKenney who hold up the fort at Kushi Institute; Devra Krassner, ND, for suggesting to me that some women with breast cancer had been helped by the macrobiotic diet; George and Judith Krassner who are living proof of that; Fern Tsao, my acupuncturist and Chinese mother; Joseph Py, D.O. for his inquisitive mind; Dixie Mills, MD and Marcel Pick, nurse practitioner, for their support at Women to Women, Yarmouth, Maine and for finding my approach credible; Ken Hamilton, MD, founder of H.O.P.E. for giving a forum for people to talk about alternative and spiritual ways of healing; for chef, Brian, at Gould Academy, for making vegan entrees available; my Oregonian friends, Heidi Peyton, Sue Stringer, and Linda Milks for their true friendship; Ellen Thomas for the menu plans; Janet Brown and Amy Rolnick, for being my friends and cooking with me; Christina Pirello for her laughter, intelligence, and creativity and taking her mother's Italian recipes and making them unique macrobiotic gems; Nancy Barstow, RN my friend and the first woman I met who healed her terminal breast cancer through macrobiotic diet and lifestyle twenty-five ago; Janet Vitt-Sommers, RN, and Hadil Kalafati, MD who I looked forward to studying with at the Kushi Institute; my friend, Debbi Gross, who taught me not to be a people pleaser; my friend, Shirley Aisha Memon, who cared and cooked for my children while I studied at the Kushi Institute; the staff at the Cancer Community Center in South Portland, Maine and to the students who attend my cooking classes—I learn as much from you as you do from me; Bill and Marie Wood for making me laugh and for organizing the Maine Macrobiotic Association; Louise Sharp for inspiring me; Judy Wohl and Jane Moriarty for their friendship and good advice; my nieces, Sarah Kelly and Kate Delaney—my cheering squad; Jacqui Morin for your hard work and keeping me organized; my life coaches, Sally McCue and Joan Borgartti, for their guidance; Nanette Crampton for getting me started with the photos, to God and the Infinite Universe for all of my learning experiences; the yin and yang of life and for bringing balance and restored health back into my life; Cheryl Richardson whose books brought me the ideas of extreme self care and learning to give up good for great; Dr. Martha Beck for "Polaris"; and last but not least Mike Joyce, CP for getting me back on two feet!

o   o   o

INTRODUCTION ○ On rare occasions, when I am drawn back to the memories of darker times, I look at a couple of photographs taken of me in 1999 when I was dying of breast cancer. I don't do this often, and several times I have considered destroying the pictures because it's hard to look at myself during those years.

In one of the photographs, I am standing with two of my sisters, Liz and Ruth. At the time the pictures were taken, I was 41 years old. I have a look on my face that's exhausted, ghost-like, and detached from reality, as if I am no longer connected to anyone or anything of this world. A wig covers my bald scalp, but is about as obvious as an ill-fitting hat. The wig is hot and my face is clammy and wan.

What the pictures don't show is my prosthetic leg, which I had been wearing since the winter of 1991, when I lost my left leg to bone cancer. Eight years later, I was diagnosed with breast cancer that had spread to my lymph nodes. As I grew weaker from the breast cancer, the artificial leg had become even more difficult to maneuver. Like my lifeless leg, my entire body was becoming too heavy for me to carry.

When these pictures were taken, I was in the midst of yet another round of chemotherapy, having already completed earlier rounds of both chemo and radiation. After this latest round of treatment, my doctor informed me as gently as she could, that I had perhaps a year to live. Other specialists were more blunt and aggressive. One told me that my only chance of survival was by undergoing a bone marrow stem cell transplant, a treatment that required extremely high doses of chemotherapy. The chemotherapy would wipe out my immune system, I was told. But the stem cells removed from my bone marrow could restore my immunity and might eventually kill the remaining cancer. As sick as I was, I somehow instinctively knew I should stay away from that approach, which scientists later discovered was worthless. Unfortunately, it had already killed thousands of women.

Still, by all accounts, I was either going to die from the disease or the treatment, or some combination of both. As my old photographs so painfully reveal, I was pretty much out of hope. Looking at those pictures now, I find it hard to believe that I was ever the woman in those pictures. Even harder to believe is that I could recover.

When it seemed that I would soon let go of this world, I was introduced to a diet and lifestyle that miraculously gave me back my health and, in a much larger sense, my life. The approach I am speaking about is macrobiotics, a diet and lifestyle whose purpose is to restore physical, emotional, and spiritual health.

Today, I am completely free of cancer. I take no drugs and undergo no form of medical treatment and I have an abundance of energy, remarkable physical strength, and a deep well of enthusiasm for life. In every respect, I am healthier and stronger than I was 20 years ago.

But macrobiotics has given me much more. Quite unexpectedly, the way of life that helped me overcome my disease also restored my relationship with my husband, Tom, which had been neglected for years. The lifestyle and philosophy opened us up to new and exciting ways of seeing life and understanding our relationship. Had I somehow survived the disease, but not changed my life, my marriage would have surely been destroyed. But the ideas that Tom and I encountered during and after my recovery transformed both of us and reanimated our love.

Before I became ill, Tom and I lived in separate and silent worlds. We were like a pair of clams on the beach, unable to share the tenderness that lived inside of us. But after my recovery, we were led through a gentle, transformative process that, in some miraculous way, caused us to open our hearts and finally connect. This is a fundamental part of my recovery. By opening my heart, my connection to my inner world—my soul—was restored.

Quite unexpectedly, my illness and recovery have given me a purpose for living. Today, I teach people how to use macrobiotics to help treat their own illnesses, especially breast cancer. I provide personal counseling in the macrobiotic way of life, teach cooking classes, and lecture on the subject of diet, health, and cancer. My life has new meaning, which, ironically, has made me more at home with all of the joys and the sorrows that are so organic to life.

A STORY AND A PRACTICAL GUIDE ○ My book is divided into two parts. Part I tells the story of my recovery. Part II is a practical guide to recovery that describes the healing diet I used to recover. I offer a month's worth of menus, and more than 100 recipes for healing breakfasts, lunches, dinners, soups, snacks, medicinal drinks, and desserts. This program can be used as an adjunct treatment for cancer. If medicine has run out of answers for you, it may still offer you the possibility of recovery. As you will see from my own story—as well as those whose stories I share in this book—many people who were given up for dead were still able to recover through the macrobiotic way of life. Anyone who suffers from cancer, and specifically breast cancer, can use this book to guide them in their macrobiotic practice.

Cancer is the most feared of all diseases. Each year, more than half a million Americans die from cancer, while 1.3 million more are diagnosed with the disease. Those numbers do not include skin cancer rates, which have multiplied so rapidly that they are no longer included in the standard cancer statistics.

For women, the most feared of all diseases, of course, is breast cancer. That fear has only increased during the last 40 years, and for good reason. In 1960, a woman's chances of getting breast cancer were 1 in 20. In the 1970s, that number jumped to 1 in 14. Today, they are 1 in 8. More than 180,000 American women are diagnosed with breast cancer each year, and nearly 40,000 die annually from the disease. According to the American Cancer Society, the estimated deaths in 2005 to breast cancer are estimated at 40,140. Given the fact that all the likely causes of breast cancer are increasing, the numbers of women who contract this terrible disease are likely to continue growing as well.

One of the reasons we are so afraid of cancer is because it seems so poorly understood by medical authorities. At least that's the message we are given. In fact, scientists know a great deal about cancer and there isn't nearly as much confusion about this illness as we are led to believe. This is especially true of breast cancer. Scientists know, for example, that a healing diet—such as the one I describe in this book—can prolong the lives of women with breast cancer. They also know the kinds of diets and lifestyles most often followed by women who contract breast cancer. In Part II of this book, I'll talk about some of the scientific evidence that supports a dietary and macrobiotic approach to cancer, and specifically breast cancer. I will show you how to understand and use macrobiotic principles to effectively use food and other healing modalities to recover from serious illness.

More and more people today are turning to macrobiotics as part of their treatment for cancer and other illnesses. Personal recovery stories, like my own, have become so well known that even the National Cancer Institute (NCI) has taken notice.

On February 25, 2002, the NCI's Cancer Advisory Panel on Alternative and Complementary Medicine (CAPCAM) voted unanimously to set aside funds to study macrobiotics as a possible treatment for cancer. The CAPCAM panel made that decision after listening to George Yu, M.D., surgeon, and professor of Urology at George Washington Medical Center, present six meticulously documented case histories of people who overcame advanced cancers with the use of the macrobiotic diet. The types of cancers that these people suffered from were malignant melanoma, pancreatic cancer, lung cancer, breast cancer, non-Hodgkins lymphoma, and endometrial cancer. All six of these people were diagnosed as "terminal" by medical doctors. All six are still alive.

Ralph Moss, Ph.D., scientist, best-selling author, and member of the NCI's CAPCAM panel, wrote the following after reading the evidence for macrobiotics and listening to Dr. Yu's testimony.:

"This session [of the CAPCAM panel] brought forth strong testimony that sometimes the adoption of a macrobiotic diet is followed by the dramatic regression of advanced cancers. A nurse told how, in 1995, she was diagnosed with lung cancer that had spread throughout her body. She received no effective conventional therapy, and reluctantly went on the macrobiotic diet. What makes this case so extraordinary is that her progress was monitored weekly by a sympathetic physician colleague. The shrinkage, and finally the disappearance, of her tumors were documented millimeter by millimeter! She has now been disease-free for over ten years."

The NCI plans to conduct a long-term study of macrobiotics as a treatment for cancer that is designated to start sometime this year.

HEALTH AFFECTS EVERY PART OF YOUR LIFE ○ Macrobiotics is more than medicine, at least as we typically think of medicine in Western terms. This way of eating can positively affect every aspect of your life. As most of us already know, there is more to health than merely the absence of negative symptoms. The emotional, psychological, and spiritual dimensions of health are what make life worth living. We naturally associate health with abundant energy, endurance, emotional stability, good appetite, deep and restful sleep, tolerance, compassion, and more frequent experiences of joy. I experienced all of these and much more as I practiced the macrobiotic approach to living. As my cancer receded and my health improved, one other experience surprised me, perhaps more than any other sign of health. That was the dramatic reduction of my fear.

Fear is the greatest impediment to our happiness and certainly our capacity to love. For most of my life, my own fears kept me trapped in restrictive and self-protective behaviors that prevented me from knowing myself or expressing who I truly am. Before I got cancer, I was living a life that others had trained me to live. I lived conventionally, and behaved as expected, because that was my training. I had been trained to eat meat, because I needed my strength. I drank milk and ate cheese because I didn't want to suffer from calcium deficiency and weak bones. I was cooperative and I tried to say the right things, because I wanted people to like me. I was respectful of authority figures, especially doctors, because they were always right. I couldn't trust my own experience or judgment, unless it was corroborated by medical tests or some other authority figure. I accepted these assumptions as facts and lived by them as if there was no other way of living. I lived by the rules, did what I was supposed to do, and by every conventional standard was a good person. Ironically, it all led me to my greatest fear—cancer. I felt betrayed, lost, angry, and terribly sad.

Macrobiotics made me see my fears in a new way. But more important, it strengthened my body and spirit so that I did not experience the same level of fear that had plagued me my entire life. This was one of the most dramatic changes I experienced as a result of my macrobiotic practice. Macrobiotics gave me a way of life that—in comparison to my previous way of living—is largely free of fear. Little did I know, but the lessening of my fear finally gave me access to my spirit.

I know, perhaps better than most that eventually I will die. But I don't want to die without giving my soul a chance to sing. That, I have found, is the basis for a truly spiritual life.

In the end, this is the greatest gift macrobiotics has given me—a chance to live more fully from my deepest and truest nature, and to gradually become the person I truly am. It can do the same for you.

PART ONE

1. In a single moment, my life is changed forever.

I lay on an x-ray table in a medical office in Portland, Oregon, waiting for the doctor to come into the room and tell me—finally—what was wrong with my left leg. The lights in the room were off, but I could see the doctor through some glass windows in an adjoining office as he examined my x-rays on a lighted view box. He studied the films with intense interest for several minutes. Soon, he called another male doctor into the room. The two exchanged a few words that I couldn't hear as one of them held up a pencil to the x-rays and used it as a pointer. He motioned with the pencil to create an invisible circle around a particular area of the x-ray. Both men studied the photograph with the same intense, scientific concentration.

That's not good, I told myself. *Something is wrong.*

The hospital gown that I was wearing was loosely tied in the back and barely covered my upper body. I was cold, exposed, and vulnerable. The x-ray table was hard and unforgiving and my left leg throbbed with pain. I wanted my clothes back so that I could cover myself. *What's taking them so long*, I wondered. The two conversed at length, apparently oblivious to my presence in the adjoining room.

It was the summer of 1988. I was 31 years old and had been experiencing discomfort in the back of my left knee for the previous six years. In the early stages, the knee was merely stiff. But over the years, it felt more and more like I had a tennis ball lodged behind my knee that prevented me from fully bending my leg. The image that kept coming to mind was having a ball stuck in an open door jam, which prevented the door from swinging closed. Gradually, the loss of motion was accompanied by increasing pain. Lately, the pain had become unbearable. I could no longer carry my 20-month old son around the house for very long before I was forced to take non-prescription pain killers and rest my leg.

During the previous six years, doctor after doctor had informed me that there was nothing wrong with my leg. One doctor was so patronizing and angry at me for taking up his time that he essentially dismissed me from his office and made it clear that I should not come back. Some part of me felt stupid and ashamed that I was bothering such an important man with my problem. But the pain and loss of motion forced me to continue to seek medical help. Perhaps I had arthritis in my knee, I told myself.

Now, as I watched the two men discuss my x-rays, I was suddenly overcome with an intense fear. Was it my imagination or did these men seem especially grave as they examined my films? One of the doctors was speaking now; the other was nodding his head in agreement. Finally, the physician who had taken my x-rays switched off the lighted view box, looked down toward the floor, and headed out of the office and toward the room in which I lay. Instinctively, I braced myself, terrified by the unstoppable force that was heading right at me.

THE PATTERNS AND CLUES WERE ALWAYS LURKING ○ I was born in 1957 and raised in Westbrook, Maine, a small town just outside of Portland, the second of five children — four girls and one boy. My mother, Dolores Bettez, was of French ancestry and was born and raised in a section of Westbrook known as Frenchtown, so named because it was inhabited by French-speaking Americans. Frenchtown was an insulated little village where we knew everyone and everyone knew us.

My mother was the hub of the family and its primary source of inspiration. We didn't have much money, but we never seemed to lack for anything. That was my mother's doing. My mother loved to play with us and often took us on outings just for fun. She was always baking cookies, brioches, and popovers, or making some beautiful meal that thrilled us when it was set upon the table. Everything she did, she did to perfection. It didn't matter whether she was washing the floor or making a Thanksgiving dinner, my mother attended to every detail with the commitment of a great manager. In another life, she would have been the head nurse of a large hospital. But in this life, she was held back — or perhaps she held herself back — by her training and her fears.

Both of my mother's parents died when she was young — her father when she was six, her mother when she was 14. Orphaned, she was raised by her sister, who was 20 years her senior. Her sister wielded her authority over my mother, and the two competed with each other for the rest of their lives. During the summer, our extended family — aunts, uncles, and cousins — often gathered at Sebago Lake for family picnics. My mother would produce the most exquisite desserts that were celebrated by the entire family. When she opened the boxes and bags that held her treasures, she would be surrounded by everyone like a flock of pigeons around a generous soul with a loaf of bread. Everything she had baked would be gone inside of an hour. Her sister's desserts, by contrast, were dull and largely ignored, a fact that gave my mother a rich, secret pleasure. As we drove home, my mother would gloat about her victory, though she always tried to hide it. She couldn't help herself. Once I asked her why she competed with my aunt. She heaved a long sigh and, with a hint of regret, admitted, that it was hard being raised by her sister. That was all she would ever say.

The loss of both her parents at such a young age instilled a host of nameless fears and insecurities in my mother. Safety was paramount in her mind. She never wanted us to venture beyond a certain distance from our house. It was as if she had erected a safe perimeter, within which she believed she could protect her family. Somehow she managed to communicate that beyond the boundaries of Westbrook lay dangers that were vague and terrifying. Hence, we clung to her out of our need for love and safety.

My father, J. Mark DeCoste, was, and still is, kind, gentle, and a highly intelligent man. He attended Bates College in Maine for two years, but had to drop out of school because his family could no longer afford the tuition. When I was a child, I felt that my father was burdened by something that I couldn't figure out. Even today, his soft, blue eyes seem distant and preoccupied with thoughts he doesn't share. In many respects, he was my mother's opposite. While she was dynamic and out-going, he was passive and introverted. He never found the work for which he had a passion. My mother was an executive secretary at the S.D. Warren Paper in Westbrook, a large paper mill that was our town's biggest employer. In the 1950s, she got my father a job at the mill where he remained until he retired in the mid-1980s.

My father loved us deeply and regularly found ways to show us that love. He took us on car rides with our grandparents to the ocean, which he loved, and down to the Portland pier to look at the ships that were in port. He enjoyed taking us on errands around town, too, especially to Vallee's Drugstore, which had an old fashion soda fountain that would dispense the most amazing ice cream sundaes and banana splits.

Like my mother, my father seemed beset with his own unspoken fears, though he dealt with them in exactly the opposite way from her. While she was gregarious and sometimes controlling, he was introverted, withdrawn, and in some way playing life safe. He sought his answers in the Catholic Church and clung tenaciously—and unquestioningly— to its dogma.

Within the safe cocoon of my family, beliefs and fears were expressed more by my parents' behaviors and the subtext of what was said, rather than by the words themselves. It was almost as if our parents gave us beliefs without ever being aware of what they were passing on to us. But in this way, they unconsciously indoctrinated us into the family's way of thinking, which in many ways proved even more powerful than our genes.

Among those beliefs was the choice of careers that were appropriate for us. My mother made it clear that the three professions that her daughters could pursue were secretary, school teacher, and nurse. (My brother was free to choose his own path, apparently.) She approved of these jobs, she said, because they provided a woman with regular hours and security.

As a child, I was not attracted to any of these professions. Instead, I was blessed with artistic talent that surfaced early in life. I could draw and paint and create interesting sculptures. Unfortunately, my mother's brother had been an artist and never made much of a living. Thus, the die was cast. To become an artist meant a life of financial hardship and failure. That was out of the question. My mother wouldn't have that for one of her children.

But there were more subtle reasons for the careers she wanted her daughters to pursue. Artists live outside the conventional boxes. They are free-thinking people and often bohemian, which on some level was frightening to my mother for its potential immorality. Being a nurse, teacher, or secretary were positions that were appropriate for a "proper lady," a term that turned up periodically and was loaded with obvious and subtle meanings.

Such beliefs were reinforced by our guilt-ridden Catholic School education. Occasionally, when I was being mischievous and managed to hurt myself, my mother would say "God punished you." I was never sure why God might punish me, or what I did to deserve punishment. But her words were consistent with my religious education, which led me to the inescapable conclusion that I wasn't good enough to deserve God's love and approval. Striving for love—whether it was God's or anyone else's—became a core characteristic of my inner life. I learned that I had to "grow" to be a "good person," the flip side of which meant that I wasn't.

The love of our family, the security it provided us, and the vague fears that lay at its roots combined to create turbulent currents and conflicting energies that manifested within me as a series of bizarre physical disorders that afflicted me during my adolescence and teenage years.

At nine, I suffered from chronic leg cramps that were so painful that they woke me in the middle of the night. My mother placed me in the bath and rubbed my legs down with hot water until the pain subsided. As a young teenager, I had menstrual cramps that caused me to double over in pain. At first, the doctor put me on Darvon and eventually Percodan, a narcotic pain reliever, but it wasn't until I was 17, when he had me take the birth control pill, that the cramps finally subsided. I remained on the Pill until I was 24.

When I was in high school, I got heart palpitations and tachycardia, or racing heartbeat. Sometimes my heart rate would suddenly accelerate to 140 beats per minute and stay there for days. My doctor gave me a mild tranquilizer, known as Atarax, which brought down my heart rate. At 18, I got psoriasis from the neck down. The condition was so severe that I was given cortisone tablets and made to take tar baths. Today, I shudder to think how toxic the tar baths and medication likely were, and wonder what, if any, role they played in my fate. Following the psoriasis, I got colitis and experienced bouts of bloody stools, which terrified me. I kept the problem to myself and eventually it went away.

After high school, I was trained as a licensed practical nurse (LPN) at Southern Main Vocational Technical College, located just two towns over in South Portland. Following graduation, I worked evenings on the orthopedic ward at Trinity Hospital. I loved the work and the people I treated.

Nursing inspired me. I attended many educational programs and one year later I decided to become a registered nurse (RN). I passed the entrance exams and was accepted into an accelerated RN program that would allow me to obtain a degree in twelve months. The school was located in New Hampshire, only three hours from my home, but once I moved into the dormitory, I quickly became homesick and suffered panic attacks that kept me awake at night and exhausted during the day. I was 21 years old, I said to myself—you're too old to be homesick. Those words didn't change anything, however. I was too ashamed by the problem to ask anyone for help, so instead I decided to leave school. I rationalized it by telling myself that I really didn't want to be a nurse. Not surprisingly, the experience left a mark on me, and revealed the deep fears I had about leaving the safety of my family, and especially my mother. But it also showed me how fear could rob me of the courage to follow my own path, and to become the person I really longed to be. I didn't realize it then, but that fear would eventually rise again, at the crossroads between life and death.

HELP WAS OFFERED, BUT I COULDN'T SEE ○ In December 1980, when I was 23, I met my future husband, Tom Wolff. Tom lived in Holyoke, Massachusetts, and often came to Maine to visit friends from his alma mater, the University of Massachusetts at Amherst. We met at a party where I had expected to meet people who turned out to be Tom's friends. As

Tom liked to put it, "You came to meet Frank and Quinny [two of Tom's friends] and got stuck with me." Part of Tom's way of courting me was to write hilarious letters that would leave me doubled over with laughter.

Tom is six-feet-five-inches tall and lean. He ran cross country in high school and has been a runner ever since. Blessed with a strong desire to be of service to others, he has always found ways to fulfill that need. When we met, he was a social worker who assisted mentally-handicapped adults. He loved it and had no ambitions to change his occupation, but his friends worked in Maine for Nike, the sports shoe manufacturer, and got him to apply, if for no other reason than to be closer to me. Tom showed up for the interview in a borrowed sports jacket and was hired on the spot.

Tom is good at everything he does and it wasn't long before the people at Nike realized what they had in him. He moved up the ladder rapidly and in January 1982 Nike made him a manager and sent him to South Korea. Despite my fears about wandering too far from my family, we were in love and already planned to marry, so I visited Tom in Korea. It looked like heaven to me, as did much of the rest of the world. We married in August of that year and immediately went to Korea, where we would live for the next three years.

Just before I left the U.S., I took a 30-mile bike ride with a friend. When I got home, the area behind my left knee was swollen and ached for a few days. I took some pain killers and dismissed the discomfort as the consequence of too much exercise.

Korea was, in all respects, the other side of the world. Years later, I would realize that the Korean people were trying to teach me advanced lessons for living, but I was too indoctrinated in the Western way of thinking to see the gifts they were offering me. The great lesson they were trying to teach me, of course, was how to take care of my health. Whenever I visited the home of one of my many Korean friends, they would put food in front of me and say, "Have some of this. It's good for your liver." Or, "Have this vegetable it's good for your digestion." "This is good for your kidneys and bones," a friend would say.

I wasn't able to make the connection between food and health that the Koreans took for granted. I believed that I was healthy and didn't need their home remedies or folk medicine. In my mind, health was a static state, something that you either have or you didn't have. I was also blinded by the Western arrogance that made me believe that, as an American, I was more sophisticated than these Asian people. I went to my doctor for health care, not my grocer or traditional herbalist.

The odd fact was that I respected my Korean friends immensely. Koreans are proud and well-educated people. In addition, their culture is steeped in a wisdom that was entirely foreign to me. For Koreans, the body is something that you care for and protect, which you do by eating appropriate foods and living a certain lifestyle. You don't just have health, they believe. You learn what is good for your body, and you *create* health. This tradition of self-care is common throughout Asia and is thousands of years old. Great physicians and sages came to understand the subtle effects of individual foods and herbs on the body's organs and overall health. Over the centuries and millennia, such knowledge became both a precise science and highly developed art. However, many of us in the U.S. don't know what to make such an age-old body of knowledge. So, without a direct understanding of food as medicine, I was more likely to treat the Korean self-care practices as folklore or, sometimes, even as superstition.

Still, I loved the Korean food and their dining customs, such as the way the food was displayed and the way Koreans sat on cushions at low tables. But as American "expats," my friends and I craved our typical American foods, such as hamburgers, pizza, bread, and especially ice cream, which soothed our occasional bouts of homesickness. There were times, of course, when American junk food wasn't available at the local market, so we turned to the black market, where we paid three times the price for Oreo cookies, Coca Cola, potato chips, pastries, and the like.

Despite my inability to embrace the wisdom of my Korean friends, I never forgot my encounter with it. Years later, it would come back to me and help save my life.

In the spring of 1984, while we were still living in Korea, I joined Chuck and Irene Hayward, who were friends of Tom's parents, on a four-day visit to Japan. The trip was intended to be a light vacation for me, but it turned out to be anything but.

On the first night I was there, I went to my hotel and was approached by an obnoxious, middle-aged American who harassed me and made sexual advances toward me. He was so persistent that I feared I might have to call the police to ward him off. The experience was unsettling, but I tried to shake it off and enjoy the rest of the trip.

The next day, the Hayward's and I visited a Shinto shrine in Kyoto. We entered the grounds by walking through tall red gates. As we made our way to the temple, a man approached us carrying a box of scrolls in his arms. Each scroll, when unraveled, revealed a series of Japanese symbols that purportedly foretold your future. The idea was that you choose a particular scroll and then had it read and interpreted by the man carrying the box. Thinking that it would be fun, the Hayward's each took a scroll and then handed it to the man who divined their future in light and entertaining ways. When he was finished with them, I choose a scroll and handed it to the man. Suddenly, he became deadly serious. He looked me in the eye and said, "Misfortune."

"What?" I said, trying to regain my balance.

"Misfortune," he said again with that same direct, penetrating look. I was reeling.

The man started to talk about ways that I could avoid misfortune, but in my haze I could barely make out the fact that he was speaking. It was as if the molecules of my body had momentarily been scattered and were now struggling to coalesce into a solid form again.

Mr. and Mrs. Hayward could feel the intensity of the moment as well. Both saw how much the man's words had upset me. Mr. Hayward tried to lighten the moment by making a joke. After a few moments, we tried to collect ourselves and put the event behind us. We continued our tour of the shrine, but whatever happened on those grounds stuck with me, even as I flew back to Korea and Tom. Once home, I explained to Tom what had happened at the Shinto Shrine.

"Meg, it's just superstition," he told me. "Don't worry about it."

"It felt real to me," I said. "Something in the way the guy said 'misfortune' to me. It hit me hard." I was obviously upset, but Tom dismissed my concerns. I was being ridiculous, as far as he was concerned. It's meaningless superstition, Tom insisted. But for me, it felt very real.

I didn't have the words to say that perhaps this man's words touched a deep chord in me and opened up a dark chamber in me, a place where I kept my deepest fears, and those of my family. This man may even have spoken words that I believed about myself, and about my future. He may have simply articulated the very belief I had about my life and my fate. But I could say none of that, because I didn't know how.

Instead, I was left to cope with the turmoil inside myself, without any way of making that turmoil legitimate or meaningful.

Events like these made me see myself as weak and needy. Tom was inherently practical and grounded, while I was becoming worrywart, or so it seemed. He was the doer, I was the feeler. That dichotomy sometimes left me feeling inadequate and inferior.

What had happened to us? I sometimes wondered. When Tom courted me, he wrote beautiful love letters. We engaged in intimate conversations that I thought would go on for as long as we lived. But once we were married, Tom focused exclusively on the practical matters of work, money, and our daily activities, while I was left to deal with all the unspoken emotions that occurred in me, and perhaps in both of us. Tom denied feeling any of the emotions or needs for closeness that I was experiencing, however. And increasingly, he saw my emotional needs as obsessive. What good would it do to talk about our anger? he would ask. Why bother going into our fears?

What made matters even worse was that I didn't understand myself. Nor did I have the vocabulary to know that, in fact, I was asking for a greater understanding of myself and of him, though at the time neither of us saw it that way. But without a deeper understanding of myself, and of life itself, I was left to flounder around in my own emotional turmoil, which at times made me look and feel like a weakling. By contrast, Tom seemed increasingly competent and mature. After awhile, I came to believe that Tom must be right. I have to become less emotional, less in need of intimate conversation—in short, more like him.

After three years in Korea, we moved to Portland, Oregon, and then to Massachusetts, and then back to Oregon. In the interim, we had our first child, Francis, in 1986. Over the years, my leg got worse. At first, I thought I might have phlebitis, but when I suggested this to a doctor he looked at me with irritation and then informed me that I had not been trained to diagnose myself. He examined my knee and told me there was nothing wrong with me. He could x-ray it, he said, but his technician was on vacation. And then he got up from his chair to indicate that our meeting was over.

Other doctors I consulted were more polite, but no more concerned with my leg than he was. Until finally, the leg became so painful that it woke me up at night. I knew I had to see someone and, if necessary, demand as much diagnostic testing as was needed to find an answer.

All of which brought me to this Portland, Oregon, medical office in the summer of 1988, where the doctor who had just examined the x-rays of my left knee was about to announce my fate.

EVERYTHING CHANGES ○ The doctor entered the room, turned on the light, and introduced himself.

"I am 98 percent sure that you have bone cancer," he said to me as I lay on the hard x-ray table. His words were too shocking for me to grasp initially.

"Couldn't I have some form of calcification behind my knee that looks on the x-ray like a tumor?" I asked.

"No, I don't believe that's the case," he said. "You've got a big tumor, the size of a lemon, in the back of your knee." He began to speak about the possibility of a long-term illness. As he spoke, it occurred to me that he looked like Charles Bronson, who starred in a series of movies called "Death Wish." He had narrow eyes that formed dark slits in his square head.

He was tough and unyielding, though I sensed that he was showing me his kinder side. Later, Tom and I referred to him as Dr. Doom.

"You'll have to have the mass biopsied," he said. He then recommended a surgeon that I should see.

I got dressed and left the office and managed to find my way to a public telephone where I called Tom and told him what had happened. By this time, I was so deep in shock that I don't recall a single word of the conversation. All I could think of was the movie, "Love Story," in which Ali McGraw plays a young college-aged woman who is in love and has all this joy to look forward to and then gets cancer and dies.

After Dr. Doom made his pronouncement, Tom and I began going out to lunch more so that we could talk about what might lay ahead. Tom was completely supportive of me and I loved the intimacy that we shared in the face of so much fear. What an irony, I thought at the time. Tragedy strikes and all of a sudden we are experiencing greater closeness and love than we do when times were good.

"Am I going to lose my leg, Tom?" I asked him one day over lunch at a cafeteria-style restaurant.

"No, Meg," he assured me. "They don't do those kinds of things in this day and age. They've got other things they can do now." Oregon, as most everyone knows, is overcast and rainy most of the year. That day was no different, but in the midst of such darkness, Tom was my light.

The physician to whom I was referred was Dr. Robert Gray, an orthopedic surgeon who specialized in bone cancer. His large office was simple and unpretentious, like the man himself. He was in his late 40s, supportive, caring, and friendly—a welcome contrast to so many of the doctors I had encountered before. Dr. Gray examined my knee and the x-rays. He then listened carefully to me as I described my long history of discomfort and pain. When I was finished, he said that it might not be as bad as I had been led to believe.

"This could be a big benign tumor," he said. He called it an osteochondroma. The reason for his optimism, he said, was that I had been suffering for many years, a fact that suggested that the tumor was slow growing. If that was the case, it might not be a malignant bone cancer, which typically grows much more rapidly than my experience suggested. His words hit Tom and me like great beams of sunlight that suddenly appeared from behind a dark and ominous cloud. Oh my God, I thought. This could be benign! We might escape this hell that we're in.

Dr. Gray did a biopsy of the tumor and sent tissue samples to a renowned pathologist in California. We had to wait a couple of weeks, but the report came back negative: the tumor was benign. Relief doesn't come close to describing how we felt. Somehow, I dodged the bullet that might have killed me.

Dr. Gray immediately made plans to remove the tumor from my leg. The shape of the growth wasn't simply round, but rather a ball in the back of my knee with finger-like projections that wrapped around the front of my knee. Before he did the operation, Dr. Gray explained that he would remove the ball itself, but would have to leave the projections behind because he would have to cut the back and the front and weaken the leg too much.

The operation was performed, and Dr. Gray removed the tumor from the back of my knee. He made a long incision along the back of my leg, from well up on the hamstring to well down along the calf. When the scar healed, it looked like a long worm had embedded itself in my leg. Dr. Gray referred to the changes the skin underwent to create this scar tissue as "keloiding."

After I had recovered from the surgery, I had the full range of movement in my leg. Soon, my leg was strong again, as well, which thrilled me. Weeks after the surgery, Dr. Gray and I discussed my rehabilitation process. During that meeting, I asked, "Is there any chance that the little tumors that are still in my leg could become malignant, Dr. Gray?"

"There's only a one percent chance of the benign tumors turning into malignancies," he said. "I'm only one percent worried," he added with a smile.

One percent, I said to myself. That means there's not much of a chance. I was relieved.

In the weeks that followed, I tried to look at the bright side of my situation. I was out of the woods, had no pain and had full use of my leg again. I was in the clear. Stay positive, I told myself. Everything worked out fine.

We lived in Lake Oswego, an affluent suburb of Portland, Oregon, a place that might have served as a poster for the American dream. Many of those who lived there were young and successful. It seemed from the outside that we had everything we had ever dreamed of, or could want. We had achieved the American dream. But at my very core was a dark fear that it all could be taken away in a single breath.

One of our neighbors was a young surgeon. Jim was so relaxed and unpretentious that Tom and I referred to him as the non-doctor-doctor.

One day, when I saw Jim in his frontyard, I walked over and asked him, "Is there any chance that benign tumors can become malignant?"

"It's possible," he said, "but not probable."

I walked away with an odd and paradoxical feeling. On one hand, I was comforted by the odds, but deep inside Jim's equivocal answer disturbed me. It wasn't just fear that I was experiencing, but something more elusive that I couldn't quite express. Whatever it was, it pressed itself against the walls of my consciousness, trying to get me to express what I couldn't quite grasp. Years later, I would realize what was attempting to make itself known to me. It was a question, based on an ancient wisdom that was arising from my cells. The question was this: Is there anything in my behavior that might determine whether those tumors remain in their benign state or are transformed into a malignant cancer? If so, than do I have the power to protect myself by acting wisely?

I could not make those insights conscious at the time. Instead, they haunted me, like a dream that I knew was important, but couldn't quite remember.

"Possible, but not probable," Jim had said. Why could I find no comfort in those words?

2. Losing my leg.

It's the safety at the center of the American dream that makes it so alluring. We have these very powerful images of the happy family, the beautiful house, and the nice cars that serve as symbols and goals for which we're supposed to strive. But it's the happy ease at the core of these images that pulls us in and makes us devote our lives to their fulfillment. Nothing bad happens to the people in those images; their lives are free of tragedy. And the message is that if you achieve those images—the happy family, the house, the cars—you'll be insulated from the unexpected. The secret power at the heart of the American dream is the promise of security.

I had all the images, but none of the peace. Fear that my cancer might return still beset me, despite Dr. Gray's assurances and the apparently successful surgery. I dealt with those fears in the only way I knew how, by devoting myself to my family and the security of its rhythms. I got up in the morning, dressed and fed my son, Francis, and got him off to pre-school by 8:30 a.m. Tom was an early riser. He had been up hours before, had gone for a nine-or-ten-mile run, showered, and headed off for work. After I dropped Francis at pre-school, I went to the health club and swam laps for about 45 minutes. I then ran errands, picked up Francis, brought him home, and gave him lunch. After lunch, I put him down for a nap. That was a relaxing part of the day. It was the one hour I had to myself before my son would be up and refreshed and ready for me to take him to the playground. I read a book or a magazine and drank a cup of mocha coffee to recharge. Sometimes I would call my mother. Whenever she asked how I was feeling, I assured her that I was fine and that everything was back to normal. *Normal.* The utter blandness of the life that word conjured up made it beautiful. Normal was synonymous with routine, with uneventful, with safe. Normal meant that I was in control, that I was safely ensconced in the life I was supposed to be living.

Later, I made dinner, a chore I distinctly disliked. I hated to cook, mostly because I never knew what to make. What do I make tonight? It was a perpetual and perplexing question before me.

We ate a regimen that included some whole grains, such as brown rice, and fresh vegetables, and just about everything else in the standard American diet. Oregonians are ecologically and nutritionally aware, so like my neighbors, I recycled and even used cloth diapers, because they were environmentally friendly. All of this politically correct behavior gave us a sense that we were doing the right thing, and perhaps gave us some reassurance against the secret fear of the unexpected. But I was still addicted to sugar and junk food. It was just that I also ate a lot of foods that I now believed to be good for me. Still, you couldn't improve your diet or recycle without learning something of the substance behind the behaviors. My understanding of nutrition, at least back then, did not go very deep. I was just starting to make vague connections between food and health.

Tom got home between 6 and 7 p.m. I accepted his long day because he was moving up in his career and making a very good living for the family. At night, we went for walks, or watched television, or read our books, or read to Francis, and put him to bed, and then went to bed ourselves.

On May 10, 1990, I gave birth to our beautiful daughter, Katherine Camille, whom we call Cammie. It was a joyful time, and I remember thinking that this was as good as life gets. Our new child added a whole new set of routines—nursing, diapers, and taking care of her every need—that gave me the deepest sense of satisfaction and grounded us all in family life. Normal. This is what life was supposed to be, at least according to all that I had been taught. But in the background of my life—and specifically in the back of my left knee—lay the small embers of fear.

That fear made me hypervigilant for any symptom that might arise in my leg. For two years after the surgery, nothing problematic arose. I enjoyed full range of motion in my leg and felt no pain. But in the fall of 1990, I started to experience small twinges of activity in my knee that my gut told me weren't right. At first, they felt like small sparks of life, followed by gnawing sensations in the bone itself. These twinges appeared sporadically. But then they became more persistent, especially while I was driving. I told my girlfriend about them and after I finished talking, she urged me to tell my doctor immediately. The reason she was so adamant was because I was speaking with so much fear. Soon I became so alarmed by the consistency of the symptoms that I called Dr. Gray and told him that I would like to have the tiny tumors that he had left behind removed from my leg. He agreed that we should take them out. He also said that given the symptoms that I described, we should have the tumors biopsied to see if they were malignant.

In October, Dr. Gray removed the remaining tumors and sent them to California for analysis. A few weeks later, we had our answer.

DARKNESS FALLS ○ One day in mid-October, Dr. Gray telephoned to tell me the results. However, the line was busy, so he called Tom at work. Tom was in the middle of a meeting, but upon being told that Dr. Gray was on the line, came to the phone immediately. Dr. Gray told Tom that the tumors were malignant.

"What do we do?" Tom asked.

"We're going to have to remove her leg," Dr. Gray replied. He then told Tom to bring me to Dr. Gray's office immediately.

Tom cried much of the way home. He was overcome with fear that I might die of the cancer. To distract himself, he turned on the radio and heard Tom Petty sing "Free Falling." "She's a good girl," Tom Petty sang, "loves her mama, loves Jesus and America, too." As Tom listened to the song it struck him how much the lyrics described me.

When he entered the house, I was sitting on the couch and was immediately surprised to see him home in the afternoon. The question popped into my mind: Did he get promoted? No, I said to myself. He doesn't look happy. Maybe he got fired.

"What's wrong?" I asked as he sat down next to me. Tom held me in his arms for a moment and then said, "We have to go to Dr. Gray's office. He got the pathology report back. The cancer is malignant." I was too stunned to talk—or to remember anything that I might have said. I got up from the couch and called a friend to come over and take care of my children while I went to the doctor. The shock enveloped me like an ever-thickening fog. The next thing I knew, Tom and I were walking into Dr. Gray's waiting room, but as soon as the receptionist saw us, we were ushered into his office. We were treated like family members, I thought.

Dr. Gray got up from his desk and came over to us. He showed us to a sitting area and the three of us sat in chairs in the middle of the room. Dr. Gray explained that the tumors in my leg were malignant and that my leg would have to be amputated in order to keep the cancer from spreading. Otherwise, there was a chance it would eventually spread to vital organs and kill me. He went on to explain that he would have to remove my leg above the knee, "Just above the flare of the condyle."

"Other doctors might try to convince you to have an operation to remove those tumors and save the leg," Dr. Gray said. "You could try to do that, but I'm convinced that eventually we would have to take the leg. There's too much risk of having the cancer spread. I've seen slower-growing tumors become full blown sarcomas."

He felt that since the cancer was still localized, my life could be protected by removing the leg. With the surgery, I had a 90 percent chance of a cure, which meant that the cancer would not re-emerge somewhere else.

"This is a failure surgery for me," Dr. Gray said. As he spoke, he started to cry. Tom also began crying, too.

"You guys," I said. "Don't worry. Everything's going to be okay. Really, it's going to be fine."

Looking back at that moment, and my words, I am appalled by my denial of my own pain and by my feeble attempt at assuaging the suffering of the two men. Again my childhood training played out, this time in that room, like some derivation of a Christian tragedy in which the person who is going to the gallows soothes those who mourn.

Dr. Gray recommended against chemotherapy. "The chemo would kill you faster than the cancer," he said. And if it didn't kill me, it might trigger another cancer 20 years from now, he warned.

"What might have caused my benign tumors to become malignant, Dr. Gray?" I asked.

"The cause is unknown, Meg," he said.

A single thought preoccupied me. How am I going to tell my son? I kept asking myself. How will this affect him? Thoughts of my little boy made the pain more intense and real. I was sinking now. My gut told me that everything was not okay, nor would it be okay simply because I had spoken those words.

The meeting with Dr. Gray took about 45 minutes, at least that's what Tom would tell me years later. When we finished talking, Dr. Gray put his arm around me as we headed toward the door. To this day, I have this clear visual image of me in my green coat with Dr. Gray's arm around me. In my mind's eye, I can even glimpse my slumped posture and vacant, shell-shocked expression.

The surgery was scheduled for late November, a month away. It was a horrible month. We were scheduled to go to Hawaii on vacation, but I had no desire to travel. I am told that many people who are about to lose a leg go for long runs so that, after the surgery, they can remember what it was like to have two legs. I didn't do anything like that. I was too much in shock to play mind games with myself. All I could feel was that I was on an unstoppable train that was roaring toward a fate that terrified me.

I had to tell my son, Francis, who was now 4 years old. I just didn't know how. Tom and I sought the advice of a therapist who specialized in these kinds of issues. After an hour-long session with her, Tom and I went home to talk to Francis. The three of us sat in the family room, Francis and I on a couch and Tom in a chair close-by.

I started out by telling Francis that I had an "owie" in my leg. "You know how sometimes people get "owies" and they hurt themselves, Francis?" I said. He nodded, unsure of where all of this was going.

"Well, Mommy's got a bad "owie" in her leg," I said. "It's called cancer. The doctor is going to fix the "owie," but Mommy is going to lose her leg. The doctor has to take my leg in order to help me get well. I'm going to be all right, though. The doctor is going to give me another leg. It won't be as good, but it will be okay because I'll be able to walk."

Tom and I could see that he was upset. And then I said, "You don't have to worry because this is not going to happen to you. You're going to be fine, and so is Daddy and little Cammie. And I'll be fine too. I've just got to go to the doctor in order to be well again."

Francis started to cry. "Why?" he asked. He looked up at me, obviously in anguish.

"Because my leg got hurt and this is the only way to fix it," I said.

"Why," he said again, clearly distraught. He started shaking his head and saying, "No, no, no..." We all embraced. Francis hugged me tight and I held him, as if protecting him against life's assaults.

Eventually, he stopped crying. I observed him closely for several days, trying to detect if there were any residual effects from our talk. He seemed to bounce back beautifully, regaining his active and happy demeanor.

We were invited to someone's house for Thanksgiving dinner. Everyone was in a festive, holiday mood, but I was having trouble simply holding myself together. I wanted to cry, and run away, and escape my fate. Meanwhile, all around me was giddy talk—people having fun, as they should at such an occasion, but for me it all occurred as if in another dimension from the one in which I was living. Color seemed to be missing—I only saw vague images in yellow and brown. I walked through the day in a deep haze, disconnected from myself and everyone else. My body went through all the appropriate motions, but my spirit was curled up in a ball in some corner of my psyche, hiding from all that was about to happen.

I kept going back to my decision to go ahead with the surgery. Dr. Gray had said that there was a 90 percent chance that the amputation would keep the cancer from spreading. On the surface, that sounded good, and it even made sense to me. After all, the cancer was in my leg. Remove the leg and you remove the cancer. It all seemed simple enough. But the cancer had already done unpredictable things. The last time Dr. Gray gave me odds, he told me that there was only a one percent chance that the tumors would become malignant. Yet, they did become malignant. Now he was telling me that there was a ten percent chance that the cancer might spread to another part of my body and eventually kill me. Clearly, the odds were growing in favor of the cancer. I really didn't know how the cancer might turn up somewhere else in my body, especially after my leg had been removed. But Dr. Gray was telling me that there was a chance—apparently a very significant chance.

But what choice did I have but to go ahead with the operation? I kept asking myself. If I didn't have the leg removed, the cancer would surely spread and I would soon be dead. This seemed like my best hope of survival. Over and over, Tom and I repeated the simple logic of what I must do: the cancer is in the leg, we said. The leg was going to be removed. That meant that the cancer no longer would be in my body. We clung to that simple logic to justify our course. At least I would be alive, I told myself.

A DAY OF LOSS ○ My leg was amputated on November 28, 1990 at Capitol Hospital. We had to get up at 5 a.m. to get to the hospital by 6. Surgery was scheduled for 7:30. Tom drove along the beautiful Terwilliger Boulevard, which is guarded on both sides by stately mansions that most people dream about owning. As we drove by these beautiful homes, I remembered the many times I had walked in this beautiful neighborhood. When Tom and I first moved from South Korea to Portland, Oregon, I used to go on five mile walks in this neighborhood, known as the West Hills. As its name implies, this is high ground in Portland and the views were stunning. I would trek up these hills for about two and-a-half or three miles, and then look out over the region. From some of these vistas, you could see Mt. St. Helens and Mt. Hood, at least on clear days. The views from here stirred my soul. And on the walk back down, I would look at the beautiful homes and dream about owning a small house with a great view. All those dreams now seemed worlds away as we made our way to the hospital.

The sun was not yet up, but the sky was clear and the day would be sunny and unseasonably warm. Neither of us knew what to say. I felt trapped and suffocated, as if I was going to my own execution. Tom would say later that he marveled at how brave I was, but all I could think of was how much I wanted all of this to be over.

The night before our HMO administrator called and said that he would not pay for the operation because Dr. Gray was overqualified, and therefore too expensive, for such a simple surgery. Dr. Gray got on the phone and proceeded to rip the administrator's lungs out, metaphorically speaking, of course. After a lengthy argument, the administrator relented and agreed to cover the surgery. We vowed never to have an HMO again.

At the hospital I was given a private room, and once I was settled, a nurse gave me a sedative, and asked me to get into a hospital Johnny. Before I knew it, I was on the gurney and being wheeled to the operating room with Tom at my side, holding my hand. Tom later recalled that, "I wanted to say something profound and meaningful to Meg. I kept thinking that we're too young to be going through this."

Too quickly, we arrived at the entry doors to the operating room and a technician stopped Tom and told him that he couldn't go any further. Tom looked down at me and with tears in his eyes said, "I love you. See you in a couple of hours." His voice broke as he said those words. With that, he let go of my hand.

I was wheeled into an operating room. Intensely bright klieg lights hung from the ceiling and blinded me momentarily. I was given another drug and then an IV was inserted into my arm. The drugs made me want to talk and tell jokes to the doctors and nurses who stood nearby. As they prepared for the surgery, they talked about sports—just another day in the operating room.

Tom went back upstairs and took a walk in back of the hospital. Capitol Hospital is a huge castle-like structure that sits high on the highest point in the West Hills section of Portland. The sun was up and the day was clear and Tom looked out at the white peaks of Mount St. Helens and Mount Hood. The beauty could not take him away from all that was happening in our lives.

"That was the lowest point of my life," Tom would say later. "There were so many questions, so many unknowns. Things seemed completely out of our control. Meg had cancer and was losing her leg. We had two children. How were we going to take care of them?"

Tom wandered in back of the hospital. Suddenly, one of my dear friends, Sue Stringer, came walking up to him. Tom was surprised to see her.

"I didn't know what to do with myself," she told Tom. "I'm a wreck thinking about Meg. I had to come down here." The two of them hugged each other and cried. They talked for a few minutes, but neither knew what to say. There was no escaping the distress. Soon, Sue left and Tom came down to the waiting area just outside the operating room.

The surgery was scheduled to take only about an hour-and-a-half. It was a fairly routine procedure, but there was one aspect that required great care and skill. Once the leg was amputated, the long nerves of the thigh would be exposed at the stump. This presented a potential problem, because those nerves would be impacted by the plastic socket of the prosthetic leg. If the nerves were exposed, I would be in severe pain every time I put any weight on the prosthetic leg. Dr. Gray, who was not only experienced, but highly skilled, attempted to compensate for this problem by tucking the nerves under a fleshy portion of my thigh, thus giving them a cushion that would absorb the blows when I put my artificial foot on the ground.

Tom didn't have to wait long before Dr. Gray emerged from the operating room in his scrubs. Tom had seen Dr. Gray many times, but only in a suit. Seeing Dr. Gray in his scrubs drew Tom a step closer to the reality that lay in the operating room.

"Everything went well," Dr. Gray told Tom. Dr. Gray's manner and expression were open, light, and confident. "Do you want to see her?"

"Yes," said Tom.

"Go in," Dr. Gray said to Tom. "She's right inside."

Tom entered a holding room that served as a foyer just outside of several adjoining operating rooms. About four or five people who had just come out of surgery waited on gurneys. All were in various stages of consciousness. Tom spotted my gurney and came over to me. I had just started to re-enter consciousness. As I entered this hazy world, I immediately felt intense and stabbing pain in my leg. I wasn't sure where I was, or what had happened to me. I was in excruciating pain and I called for help and cried out in pain. I could feel people rushing over to me. Through the haze, I saw the horror on Tom's face. In order to deal with the unbearable pain, I focused my thoughts on

Tom and my children, those I loved the most, and tried to flee my body. I was given more drugs and felt myself falling away from Tom and into the darkness of sleep.

From Tom's perspective, the entire event was shocking and mystifying. "The minute I saw Meg, I could tell she was in obvious physical and mental distress," Tom later recalled. "Suddenly, she started screaming. She was bouncing off the gurney, she was in so much pain. Dr. Gray ran into the room and he and a nurse administered more drugs and pretty soon she was out again. Dr. Gray asked me to leave the room, and I went back outside to the waiting room. I tried to collect myself. I knew immediately that I should never have been in there. Or at least, I should never have been sent in there after being led to believe that it would be so different from how it was. Dr. Gray seemed so sure that everything was under control and Meg was basically okay. But she was anything but. Later, he explained that the spinal anesthesia wore off too quickly.

"It was like the difference between a war movie and a real war." Tom later said. "In the movies, men get shot, they fall down, and it's all pretty neat and clean, but in real life, men get shot and they scream and there's blood and gore and there's nothing neat about any of it. Well, this was pretty much the same thing. Dr. Gray led me to think that I was going in to visit my wife and that it would be a comforting moment. He said that everything had gone well. And then I go in there and everything is out of control and Meg's in all this pain.

"In retrospect, I realize now that all of this was a metaphor for how things would unfold in the months and years ahead. The doctors acted so sure, as if everything was under control, and then everything went very differently from what we had been told."

The doctors kept me drugged that day and I spent the night in the hospital, sleeping. The next day I woke up from surgery and realized that my leg was gone. It's over, I told myself. But, it was just beginning.

3. An artificial leg, a drifting marriage.

When I was a child, my friends and I would often play at the railroad tracks near our house and I would return home with my feet black with tar. My mother never wanted us to go near the railroad tracks—the thought of us being down there terrified her, as it would any parent. But there was a strange quality and mystery about those tracks that drew me to them. Perhaps it was the rails that ran to the unknown, or the courage of trains that hurtled into the night. Whenever I came home with black feet, my mother knew where I'd been and would scold me. But, that never stopped me from going back. In the summer I hated wearing my shoes, which meant that my feet were often black.

Now my left foot and most of my left leg, were gone. And the entire world was different. Until you lose your foot, you don't realize how much it pulls you into your body and connects you to the earth. My feet were more than flat surfaces on a flat earth. They grabbed hold of the ground and felt its security. My feet signaled my brain that they had made contact with the most secure part of life. Now the ground was gone, at least on one side of my body, and with it my connection to the earth. Somehow, life was less real.

I could not feel my body in the same way, either. I couldn't be as fully present in my body anymore. The trauma of the surgery had caused my spirit to retreat. My body was wounded and in terrible pain, which had to be dulled by pain killers. It was almost as if my body had turned into a war zone that I no longer wanted to enter for all its pain and bloody memories. For the first few months after the surgery, I found myself wandering into deep thought. Sometimes at the dinner table, Tom would break into my new world and say, "Meg, Francis has been trying to ask you a question."

"Oh, I'm sorry, honey. What is it?" Until Tom had spoken, I had not heard a single world.

The loss of intimate contact with the physical body and the earth was especially profound because I am essentially a tactile person. When I was a child, I loved catching frogs and putting them in coffee cans. I loved handling worms, swimming, and playing in the sand. And when my feet were black with dirt or tar in the evenings, it meant that it had been a good day.

Now, the simplest activities were major challenges. Getting out of bed, going to the bathroom, and getting dressed required entirely new movements that were foreign and intensely awkward. I could no longer hold my children and walk around the house. Whenever I held Cammie, now seven months old, or Francis, now four, I had to be sitting or lying down first so that Tom could hand one or the other to me. When Francis was an infant, I would jump out of bed in the morning and take care of whatever chores needed doing before he woke up. Once he was awake, I'd nurse, bathe, and dress him, and then we'd both be off on whatever errands we had to run that day. I loved the life I had as a mother and homemaker. But all of that was gone now. In a deep recess of my mind, I knew that part of my motherhood had been lost when my leg was taken.

Many mornings, I would wake up hours before everyone else and lie in bed immobilized by depression. Part of my problem was that I suffered from insomnia and awoke physically exhausted. Night after night I would lie awake and wonder whether I had made the right decision to have my leg amputated. There seemed no other choice, but that didn't stop me from questioning the choice I had made. Memories of having two legs and being able to walk, and even run, clouded my mind. Beset by anxieties about whether I would ever feel whole again, there was no place in my mind where I could rest and relax and allow myself to fall to sleep. In the blink of an eye, it seemed, it would be 2 a.m. and I'd start worrying about whether I would get any sleep that night, which only served to keep me awake longer.

Still, for the first three months after the surgery, I often found myself returning to my bed during the day, exhausted. Finally, Tom and I hired an au pair to help with the children while I spent hours at the prosthetist and physical therapist. Tom ended up doing a lot of the chores around the house, in addition to his full day at Nike.

I needed crutches to get around, which presented another set of adjustments. On crutches, both my arms and hands were occupied. So it was impossible to perform even the simplest tasks, such as carrying a plate of food or a cup of coffee from the kitchen to the table. What was especially difficult was transporting my six month old around the house. I found myself scooting around on my bottom, pushing Cammie in her little baby carrier. This was her mode of transportation until I got my first prosthesis a few months later.

I started dreaming about my foot. In one of those dreams, I was running effortlessly. Suddenly, someone came up to me and said, "You're missing a foot." And I looked down and said, "Yeah." I also experienced phantom limb, especially when I awoke in the morning and, still half asleep, got out of bed and tried to put my foot on the floor. I could almost feel the floor below my missing foot. The daily revelation that I had no foot was intensely sad. Each day, I had to reestablish a new reality, one in which I had only one leg.

It wasn't long after I got home from the hospital that Desert Storm exploded. The 1991 U.S. and British-led invasion of Iraq seemed to heighten my sense of dread. People were dying and I lost my leg. War took center stage on the television. My life and the war seemed interwoven. The surgery had left me in a lot of pain, for which I was taking prescription pain relievers. Most days, I lay in bed and watched *CNN*, transfixed to every detail, as if its resolution might transform my own life, too.

The shock of the surgery also created seismic shifts in my body that gradually evolved into other problems. Just a few months after the surgery, I developed chronic headaches. At first, I used a variety of over-the-counter medications, but they only dulled the pain. My doctor prescribed Hismanal, an anti-histamine and cortisone spray that gave me temporary relief. When that drug was no longer effective, she prescribed Becanase, another cortisone spray for headaches. This drug relieved the pain almost instantly. Soon, I developed sinus problems that included a chronic runny nose and post-nasal drip. I attributed this to the wet and overcast weather of Portland, which gave rise to widespread mold. The sun does shine in Oregon—just not enough, especially if you're looking to dry out your house and your sinuses.

The shock of the surgery, the pain in my leg and head, my sinus trouble, and the drugs all combined to make me detached and numb. My mind wandered off into far off regions of my imagination. Out of the blue, I started to experience panic attacks. I would suddenly be unable to catch my breath and my heart would race and I'd gasp for air. Terror-stricken, I feared I might be having a heart attack or some kind of involuntary seizure.

The panic attacks resulted in another prescription. At first, the doctor prescribed Atenolol, a beta blocker that reduced my heart palpitations. Later, I took the anti-anxiety medication, Klonopin, to help me sleep, and it did provide me with a good night's rest. I also sought counseling from a therapist who helped me grieve the loss of my leg. Talking to her also made me feel safer. Gradually, the panic attacks eased and I found myself able to relax again. But I had only scratched the surface of my grief. At that point, I was still too shocked to penetrate the pain that lay within me. It would be months before I could truly hold myself with compassion and let myself express my sadness.

TO WALK AGAIN ○ I was eager to get a prosthetic leg. I thought that if I could walk again on two legs—even though one of them would be artificial—I would start to feel that my life was coming back under my own control. Dr. Gray had given me a referral for a man in Portland who made artificial limbs and six weeks after the surgery, I made an appointment with him. Before I visited the man, I had visions of a high-tech laboratory where people were fitted for their legs with scientific precision. I had seen commercials in which people played basketball and did other amazing feats on artificial legs. I was eager to be one of those people.

Instead I found an old, dilapidated building in a rundown part of town. Inside, the office was dark and covered with cheap wall paneling. The man was 60, bald, and overweight. His shirt was stained and he smelled of cigarette smoke. When I arrived, he offered me a seat in a wheel chair. I put my crutches aside and sat down.

"I've got a terrible sickness, ma'm" he told me. As he spoke, he eyed me up and down. "And my back hurts. My spine has been fused." I had no idea why he was telling me this and I didn't know what to say. "I have a lot of pain," he continued. He moved around his office hunched over, his gaze either toward the floor or on me.

"I have to take your measurements, so take your clothes off," he said. He didn't give me anything to change into, so I wiggled out of my pants and sat in my underwear.

"You'll have to stand up so I can measure your leg," he said. He got his cloth measuring tape and turned and looked at me. Something passed between us in that moment that frightened me and made me want to get out of there as quickly as I could. I held my ground, wanting so badly for this to turn out right. He measured my leg and as he touched me, my stomach turned. Once the measurements were taken, I quickly got dressed, filled out the paperwork that he had given me, signed, and fled.

One week later, I was back in his office to be fitted with my new leg. The thing was long, heavy, clumsy, and ugly. In order to put on the prosthesis, I had to undress again. He took out a large sock that he slipped over my short limb. The limb and the sock were placed inside the prosthetic socket at the top of the artificial leg. Once my short limb was in the socket, the leg was held on by a belt that was strapped around my waist.

Immediately, we both knew that the leg didn't fit.

"You must have gained weight," the man said to me.

"No, I didn't gain any weight," I said.

"Well, something's changed in your leg. It wasn't like this last week."

"I don't know," I said. "I'm not doing anything different."

"Your leg is different. That's why it's not fitting."

He made some adjustments. "It's going to take some time to get used to," he told me.

"It seems awfully heavy," I said.

"You'll get used to it," he replied.

"Can I sit on the floor," I asked? I said that I often sit on the floor to change my daughter's diapers or to play with my son.

"No, you don't sit on the floor with a prosthesis, ma'm," he said.

I went home and began wearing the artificial leg. It was clumsy, remarkably heavy, and didn't fit. Soon, it threw my back and neck out of alignment. In addition, Dr. Gray had failed to tuck one of the large nerves in my severed limb under a protective layer of flesh. The impact of my leg and the prosthesis caused tremendous pain.

No, I said to myself. This is not state of the art. There must be something better than this. Thus began a bizarre odyssey in which I hunted for a competent prosthetic limb maker. It was like searching for the Holy Grail. I'd read or hear about a specialist in Vancouver, British Columbia, or another in Seattle, Washington, or still another in San Diego. In no time, I would have an appointment with the specialist to have him create a new leg for me. I'd arrive in a city and stay in dumpy hotels for weeks on end. The prosthetist always wanted me available on short notice so that, as the leg was being constructed, he could adjust it again and again to provide the closest possible fit.

Each time I went to see a new prosthetist, I was filled with hope that this was the man who had mastered both the art and the science of prosthetics. I kept my hopes alive by telling myself that, finally, I would get a leg that would give me freedom of movement again. And every time, I would experience the same disappointment. Not only was the leg uncomfortable, heavy, and ill-fitting, but after numerous adjustments, the prosthetists blamed me for the fact that the artificial limb didn't fit. I had gained weight since he took the original measurements, or I had lost weight, or I was retaining water. After this pattern repeated itself, I realized that the world of artificial-limb makers is not made up of highly trained specialists, capable of producing a proper socket fit. Even with today's technology, the art of fitting the socket comfortably has yet to be perfected. There are many high-tech knees and feet, but these are useless with an ill-fitting socket.

The experience often brought me to tears of despair. Why couldn't I get an artificial limb that actually fit and allowed me to walk again? I kept asking. I had the finances and I was willing to go anywhere to find a person who could make a leg that fit. But the problem is more complex than just the prosthetist's talent, or lack of it. Even when a rough fit was achieved, my real leg, or what was left of it, did in fact change as I walked on the artificial leg. The body fat in my leg would melt away with exercise. Also, some muscle mass would be lost as the socket of the artificial limb wore away at my leg. Even under the best circumstances, an artificial leg that fit in January might not fit in April, which meant that I was regularly going back to the prosthetists for readjustments. Of course, I relied on my crutches, but the awkwardness of crutches forced me to do everything more slowly, and with much greater effort.

More insidious was the fact that I didn't have the energy that I used to have. Of course, even the simplest acts, such as making the bed, or getting the telephone, or answering the doorbell, required more energy than ever before. When the phone rang, for example, I would have to get my crutches, get up on them, and then hop along in a hurry before the phone stopped ringing. There was more to my loss of energy than the fact that life required more work now. The loss of my leg left my body with far less power because most of the muscle in my left leg was gone. My body was physically weaker. It had been wounded. I was more tired now than I had ever been before. There was less of me, in both body and spirit, with which to confront the world.

I never spoke about any of these things to anyone. I told myself and others that I was lucky to be alive, and I meant it. I could be far worse off, I said. I can still get around. I have my family. I am still a very fortunate woman.

I was also a much slower woman, which created problems for those around me. Even when I had two good legs, I was slower than many people, especially Tom, who could usually do the same things I did in half the time. Now I was slower than I had ever been and everything took twice the effort. I didn't want people to wait for me, or to feel that they had to make special allowances for me. I was still strong and I could keep up, I told myself. But telling myself such things didn't make it so.

SHOCK'S ERODING EFFECTS ON OUR MARRIAGE ○ Our marriage was changed in every conceivable way. Of course, the loss of my leg dramatically affected our sexual relationship. It was quite awhile before my leg had healed that we could even consider making love. Our initial attempts were awkward and emotionally painful. I felt extremely self-conscious, vulnerable, and inadequate. And I was also concerned, at least at first, that the impact of Tom's body on my residual limb might cause pain. Tom was affected nearly as much as I was.

"I was intensely self-conscious and cautious," Tom recalled years later. "There was a whole different image of Meg's body, and I felt totally vulnerable and sensitive to possibly hurting Meg. It took me a long time before I could look at her leg and not feel terrible anguish. All our movements were very careful, and there were all of these new emotions, which got in the way of any spontaneity or passion. I felt embarrassed and awkward.

"For the first nine years of our marriage, my wife had two legs and could walk, and then all of a sudden she has cancer and her leg is gone. It was terrifying to me on some level. I believed that I shouldn't talk about what I was feeling, because I didn't want to make Meg feel worse or rejected. So I pretended as best I could that everything was normal. I was trying to say that I still accept you, that I love you, but it was the worst nightmare you could imagine. And I couldn't put words to any of it."

Without any vocabulary to describe our feelings, or even the knowledge that we needed to talk about those feelings in order to keep our love alive, we settled into a kind of bunker mentality. After he got home from work at night, Tom did the chores that I hadn't gotten to that day. On any given night, he'd cook dinner, attend to the children, straighten the house, and do the laundry. And all of it riddled me with guilt. In the back of my mind, a little voice would say that I could no longer function and I wasn't beautiful anymore. What good was I? "You married a woman with two legs," I told him one night. "Now look at me. I can't get around. I can't do what I need to do. Look at what you're stuck with—me!"

"Meg, there are no guarantees in life," Tom said. And part of him meant it. He was being Tom—strong, practical, and in complete denial of all the pain that he and I were experiencing. It was a stoicism borne from denial. But there was more to the picture than understanding, or the lack of it. Both of us were suffering in ways that neither could understand nor admit. And little by little, the burdens of our circumstances made both of us angry.

Tom didn't understand what I was going through and, as strong people often do, he doubted the legitimacy of many of my complaints, which seemed endless. I often had difficulty getting out of bed in the morning; I was shocked, detached, and sometimes distant; I had leg pain and headaches, sinus trouble, and my artificial leg didn't fit. And then I'd have to travel to some distant city to have a prosthetist make me a new leg, or adjust the existing one. Whenever I left, the burdens of the family fell even heavier on Tom. When I got home, I would soon discover that the leg still wasn't fitting right. Tom was as frustrated as I was—only his frustration was with me.

"What do you mean, the leg's not right?" he wanted to know. "You just spent three weeks away trying to get the leg right." Although this question infuriated me, I had to admit that he had every right to ask it. The problem was that even I couldn't answer it.

Gradually, I got some of my strength back and did as much around the house as I could. Tom would come home at night and find the things that I hadn't been able to get to that day, like the laundry or paying the bills. He didn't accuse me of being lazy—at least not directly. He could ask a question in such a way that he immediately put me on the defensive. "You didn't do the laundry?" he'd ask. "Dinner's not ready? What have you been doing all day?"

"Cleaning the house, taking care of the kids and dragging my leg around", I retorted. Still, his accusing questions triggered my guilt—a pattern that arose from my own childhood—and made me doubt myself all the more. Of course, I could never experience guilt without experiencing anger, too, which made me even angrier at Tom.

Tom wanted to go out or have other couples over to our house on the weekends, but I was often too tired. But I was also depressed, though I did all I could to hide it. Going places was difficult for me. The more I walked on the leg, the more pain I experienced in my residual limb. And the weight and clumsiness of the leg made going anywhere difficult.

Tom also had many work-related social functions that he had to attend without me. "Some of the people at work knew something about what Meg was going through, but many didn't. I had to show up at these functions alone, and a lot of people were wondering what was going on in my marriage. It was difficult. A lot of times, I was really angry at Meg for not going with me to these events, but I never said very much about it. Like a lot of other emotions that I was experiencing, I kept it inside."

All of this would have exhausted and upset a saint. But there was an even deeper disappointment that Tom had to carry, one that he would not let himself address or speak about. He was disappointed that he had been robbed of the woman he had married. He had dreams for our marriage and family, too, and now many of those dreams appeared to be snuffed out. Tom dealt with all of this pain in the only way he knew how—he quietly did all he could to keep the ship sailing. That's what he was trained to do by his family.

Tom was the second of nine children. His parents, both strong and disciplined, raised their children to be competent and self-reliant. Each child graduated from college and upon graduation was expected to get a job and become independent. There was no room for self-pity in the Wolff household. Tom's father, Charlie, ran an office for an insurance company. A firm disciplinarian, he stressed honesty, integrity, and uprightness. Charlie came by these virtues the hard way—by being raised by a sickly mother and an absentee father. While still a boy, Charlie became the man of the house—and never stopped being the man of the house.

Everyone who knows Charlie respects him almost instantly. He has a strong bearing and his integrity and self-discipline radiate through his personality. Yet, for all his personal strength, he is also a loving father who was actively involved in his children's lives. Tom ran cross-country in high school. The meets would usually take place in the afternoons, during the workday. Yet, whenever the runner's got ready at the starting line, Tom would look over into the crowd and see his father, standing there with a stop watch and looking over at Tom as if he were the only young man running that day. As Tom would say years later, Charlie didn't know much about cross country, or about optimal times for the two-and-three-quarter mile race, but he'd be there in the crowd, stopwatch at the ready, and winking at Tom before the race began.

Tom's mother, Alice, is reserved, and every bit as strong as Charlie. You can talk to Alice about hardships, which she has known a lot of herself. Alice lost her father when she was four years old, and her mother when she was 11. Orphaned, she had to go to boarding school and be raised by nuns.

Yet, she doesn't show a trace of self-pity or bitterness. Like Charlie, Alice taught her children to look trouble in the eye and get to work.

Whenever there was a crisis in Tom's family, everyone went off to his separate corner of the house and found something positive to do. "Our family was never really intimate," Tom would say years later. When Tom was 13, his mother suffered an extended illness. Tom responded by becoming the family's short-order cook, turning out 17 hamburgers and buckets-full of French fries every night. In Tom's house, you showed appropriate concern for those who suffered, but you didn't express the pain or fear that you may have been feeling. Instead, you soldiered on by doing whatever was needed to maintain order and stability in the family. In this way, Tom became a kind of compassionate-survivor. When he graduated from college, he became a social worker and took a job working with mentally-handicapped adults. When you're one of nine children—and the oldest boy at that—social work comes naturally. So does compassion, even when you don't talk about it. One of Tom's co-workers, whose seniority made him virtually untouchable, made a habit of verbally abusing the handicapped residents with whom Tom worked. When the person refused to stop such behavior, Tom insisted that his superiors get rid of the staff member, which they did, but only after Tom testified in court against the person.

When I fell into the dark netherworld that now engulfed me, Tom didn't know what to do except to work and run—literally. Running always gave Tom solace. After I lost my leg, he decided that it was time to train for a marathon. Every morning, he'd get up around 5 a.m. and run between 10 and 15 miles before going to work at 8. On some weekend mornings, Tom would do as many as 27 miles. On one sunny morning, after he had run for hours, he sat down on a park bench and watched people stroll by. He saw a couple walking arm in arm and thought, *We would be more whole if Meg had two legs*. Many years later, he would say, "Whenever I thought about all that we were going through, I had all these conflicting feelings that I couldn't sort out. Part of me felt guilty for being able to run. Maybe I had just run 10 or 15 miles and Meg can't do that. I felt guilty about that. But I also felt that I had lost a part of me when Meg lost her leg. And maybe I was affirming to myself that I could still run. Tomorrow isn't guaranteed us. I didn't know how much longer I could run. But I knew that I had to keep running. I had to keep going, being reliable, being supportive, and doing everything that I needed to do. And I couldn't think too much about what we were going through, because I was afraid that if I thought too much about it, I would start crying and maybe I'd never stop."

SURVIVAL PATTERNS THAT FAILED TO NOURISH EITHER OF US ○ Tom was behaving in ways that he was trained to believe were strong and heroic, but I was suffering with his absence. All the pain that we were going through had closed his heart, just as it had mine. But I needed him to talk to me, to share his feelings, and to listen to mine. I was desperately in need of intimacy with him, to know that we were in this together, and that we were supporting each other and that he still loved me, even if I was less than I had been when he married me. His distance, and his anger at me, made me feel shut out from him. Looking back now, I realize that I couldn't blame him for his silence. Neither of us knew how to talk about our pain—we had both been trained to believe that we were better off denying our feelings. If anyone had asked us what we were really feeling, both of us would have said, "What good would it do to talk about our anger, our sadness, and our feelings of loss and disappointment." Little did we realize how much love, healing, and intimacy can be experienced by doing just that. We didn't know at the time that at the bottom of those feelings lay the rebirth of our marriage. Instead, we remained shut-ins within our silent worlds and, in the course of things, we drifted further and further apart.

In time, we restricted ourselves to safe but increasingly lifeless conversations. We spoke about the immediate details of our lives—our work, the children, the bills, the chores that needed doing, the material things we planned to buy. We still locked horns like angry rams from time to time, of course and we'd scream at one another at the top of our lungs. But our arguments never got past the immediate issue about which we were fighting. We never got down to the real source of our pain—that we were losing ourselves and each other.

In my dazed and fog-bound world, my heart was breaking.

4. The first cracks appear in the edifice of faith.

My mother's love flowed to us through her cooking. I think she knew this, if only instinctively, because she eschewed shortcuts. She never bought boxed cereals, for example. Instead, our breakfasts were eggs and bacon, or pancakes, or French toast, or brioches and blueberry muffins that she made from scratch. Because we lived close to school, my mother insisted that we come home each day for a hot lunch, which usually consisted of breaded fish, or steak, or baked ham with brown sugar and pineapple slices, accompanied by potatoes and vegetables. In the winter, those vegetables were usually frozen corn or peas, but in the late spring and summer, they were often fresh from her garden. Even when we were teenagers and my mother went back to work full-time, she made homemade dinners every night, which were often followed by a batch of her sugar cookies or some other wonderful dessert.

Modern life has weakened this connection between food and motherly love, in part because so many of us get our food from restaurants, or as take-out, but in our house food came from my mother. She was its source, even when it came from the grocery store. Every Thursday, my mother did her shopping, and when her car pulled up in front of our house, we ran out and playfully assaulted her and her bags of food. "You don't even let me get inside the house," she used to say, usually a little laugh playing in her voice, as the five of us tried to steal treats from the bags she carried.

At heart, my mother was two things, above all else: first, a mother and second an artist. She was devoted to her children and she had an artist's gift that emerged in the kitchen. Yes, she loved my father, and the two of them shared a very special bond. But her relationship with her children was instinctual and unconditional. Her love for us fueled her artistic gifts and gave them purpose. She stocked the kitchen with simple fare—milk, eggs, flour, bread, sugar, and various kinds of meats—that she alchemically altered into small gifts of love that we could eat.

We balanced the purity of my mother's food with the pure junk that we got at Mr. Joe Soucy's corner candy store, which was down the street from us. Every week, I got an allowance of 35 cents, most of which I spent on penny candy—mint juleps, Tootsie Rolls, hard candy, gooey sweet stuff that came inside wax Coke bottles, and Bazooka bubble gum. The penny candies used to sit in glass bins that we would point to and say, "I want two of those and five of those and five more of those." One of the great things about penny candy was their colors—reds that don't exist anywhere in nature, cobalt blues, black licorice, swirls of white and green. When you ate penny candy, you ate color—wild colors—pink, yellow, lime green, electric blue, and purple. Candy stores seemed lit by their own special light, as if the candy itself gave off a glow. No kid could resist it.

Until I was in the eighth grade, my diet was controlled primarily by my mother and Mr. Soucy. But once I got to be 15, and entered my rebellious years, the greasy kitchens of McDonalds, Burger King, Dairy Queen, and a slew of other fast food houses provided an ever-increasing number of my meals. Instead of my mother's homemade fare, I ate mass-produced hamburgers, cheeseburgers, Whoppers, and Big Macs. I drank milk shakes and sodas. And in place of my mother's garden and frozen vegetables, I ate French fries and ketchup. The one food group I ate that I thought was healthy was milk products, especially cheese and yogurt. "It's good for your bones," my mother used to say, which is ironic because my first cancer was bone cancer.

Perhaps because food was so central to our lives, I found myself mysteriously drawn to the subject of diet and health after I lost my leg. For months, all I read about was food and how it affected the body. Among the books I bought was *The Cancer Prevention Diet*, by Michio Kushi, with Alex Jack (St. Martins Press, 1988), which describes the macrobiotic diet and the macrobiotic approach to the prevention and recovery from cancer. In that book, Kushi states that bone cancer is caused by meat, eggs, and cheese. He also suggests that a macrobiotic diet could be used to help treat cancer and eliminate it from the body.

The ideas presented in *The Cancer Prevention Diet* were not altogether foreign to me. Nearly a decade earlier, when we lived in Korea, my father gave me a book entitled *Healing Miracles*, by Ball State University Professor Jean Kohler. Kohler wrote that he used a macrobiotic diet to heal himself of pancreatic cancer.

Meanwhile, I consulted a naturopathic physician, one who uses natural medicines to treat disease. He advised me to increase whole grains and vegetables, reduce meat, and eliminate dairy foods. He maintained that dairy was the source of allergies that might be causing the headaches that I chronically suffered from.

I thought that the *Cancer Prevention Diet* and Jean Kohler's book were interesting, but the information did not penetrate me very deeply. Looking back now, I realize how disconnected I was from my own inner wisdom. The Kushi and Kohler books were echoes of the ancient Asian voice, which first began calling out to me while I lived in Korea. The Koreans, Chinese, and Japanese ate very similar diets, which were based largely on grains, vegetables, beans, fruit, and small amounts of animal foods. All three cultures had developed advanced medical systems that used food as medicine. This understanding, this art, had been developed over three thousand years by physicians and sages. It was among the greatest of human accomplishments. But once again, I was standing before this awesome body of knowledge and didn't notice it.

What I did notice was food's effects on Americans. I had been out of the country for three years, and when I returned, I couldn't help but notice how many Americans were overweight, especially compared to Koreans. In Korea, the overweight person is rare, but overweight people were the norm in America. What was happening to my country? Obesity was not the only problem, I quickly learned. Many serious illnesses had increased dramatically in the 1980s and '90s. Among them were diabetes and cancer.

I didn't realize it then, but these health books, and my visits to the naturopath, were my first tentative steps on my search for an answer to cancer. I wasn't ready to connect the dots, however. The idea that food could be a form of medicine was largely lost on me. I did make small changes in diet. I included many more whole grains, such as brown rice, and lots of fresh vegetables, and I chose organic foods as often as I could. But we also ate meat and chicken, eggs and dairy foods. I developed a fondness for cheese, which I continued to eat almost daily. I only drank a little milk, but also ate yogurt and ice cream. I also drank coffee everyday, and continued to eat sugar, though in smaller quantities than before.

Still, the idea that diet was somehow related to cancer sat in my consciousness and I decided to talk to Dr. Gray the next time I saw him.

As a former cancer patient, I continued to see Dr. Gray regularly for a wide array of tests, including an annual magnetic resonance imaging (MRI) to see if there was any trace of cancer elsewhere in my body. He also monitored my blood work. At one of our meetings, I asked Dr. Gray if the typical American diet might be somehow a cause of cancer.

Dr. Gray smiled and shook his head. "Americans have the best diet in the world, Meg. There is no way that our diet causes cancer," he said. Cancer might be a caused by a virus, he said. It might even be communicable in some way. He confided that he himself worried about getting cancer after working with so many people who had it. He had even considered what he would do if he got cancer, especially bone cancer, which was his specialty. After a pause, he said that he would do exactly what I was doing—including having his leg removed, if that's where the cancer turned up.

Something very unsettling happened as I listened to Dr. Gray. I felt intuitively that everything he was saying was wrong. I don't know why I felt this, but I was aware of how uncomfortable I was with my own feelings. I had been trained throughout my life to be cooperative and compliant, especially with male authority figures. Dr. Gray was my lifeline. He was a doctor. How could I question this man? Not only did he know more than I did, but I needed him to be right about everything! But from deep inside, my gut instinct that every so often would rally in protest against words that didn't ring true, was now shouting at me that Dr. Gray was wrong." He didn't know about diet and health, my spirit was saying, even as he pretended to know. And this awareness threw me into conflict. I was emotionally upset and even a bit angry, though I didn't dare show it. I appeared agreeable and compliant—in other words, I was being a nice woman and even a good girl.

But in that moment, I was experiencing a deep conflict inside of me. Some part of my being, a part that lived in every one of my cells, knew that Dr. Gray was wrong. I don't really know how I knew—I just did. But another part of me insisted that I had no right to question a doctor, especially a male doctor. After all, I had been taught that men were the source of my physical and spiritual salvation. I had been raised a Roman Catholic and educated, until the fifth grade, at St. Hyacinth's Catholic School in Westbrook. My formative education had been shaped by priests and nuns. As vague as God was, He was a He. Next came Jesus and then came the priests. Nuns were second class citizens of the Church, handmaidens to the priests. Even as a child, I realized that men were superior to women. Why else did men celebrate the mass and give out communion—the most sacred duties of the Church—while nuns taught school and, as far as I could tell, many lived miserable lives.

Where was I on the spiritual hierarchy? Way, way down, and in the back of the classroom. My catechism had taught that I was marked from birth with original sin, a condition no one fully defined. But it was hinted at, in something of a stage whisper that original sin had to do with sex, which was the source of all kinds of trouble. Mary, the Virgin Mother, was born without original sin and didn't have sex in order to conceive Jesus. She was pure and holy. Since I was born with original sin, I was not pure and holy. Like all other girls, I was in danger of becoming more like Eve, the temptress who made Adam eat the apple. The apple, we were taught, was a symbol for sex. As a little girl, my mind assembled the puzzle pieces—it wasn't hard. Mary was born without original sin, didn't have sex, and was a saint. Eve played with the snake, had sex, and got us all tossed out of the Garden of Eden. Women were the reason we were expelled from paradise and, thus, were the root cause of all human suffering.

Original sin was not confined entirely to sex, however. It was a vague condition of evil that stained human souls and made it impossible to get to heaven without the intervention of the Church, which were the priests. The priests had the power to keep us out of hell, partly because they were celibate, I presumed. The Church meant to keep the priests safe from women, otherwise there was no hope of redemption.

In my family, Church and religion were synonymous with sacrifice and guilt. My parents went to church on Sundays, and later Saturday night, when Vatican II decided to move the Sabbath. St. Hyacinth's Church, a massive and beautiful building, sat in the middle of Frenchtown, a village comprised of poor people, among them my parents. My mother and father gave whatever they could when the collection plate came around every Sunday, or Saturday night.

My mother's mother gave more than money. She had lost a child many years before my mother was born. Her second child was a boy, but while still an infant, he became dangerously ill. Desperate to save his life, my grandmother promised God that if he spared her son, she would see that he became a priest. He survived, and at the age of 13, was shipped off to the seminary to he raised by priests—and become one himself. It was widely believed within the Church that if a mother raised a son to become a priest, the mother would get special consideration when God decided if she would go to heaven. Presumably, my Uncle Gene, the priest, helped save his mother's soul.

The heavy yoke of the Church shaped the character and behavior of those around me. Going to Church with some of my extended family members was like witnessing a production of staged religious fervor. What a strange repulsion I felt when I watched my cousins pray with pride and make a show of their rosaries and piousness. Their religious fervor made them subtly divisive, as if they were part of the ultimate club whose membership guaranteed them God's love. Being a part of such a club did not make them more compassionate or understanding of others. On the contrary, it seemed that they could only feel good about themselves by criticizing others. Of course, in their eyes, I was hopeless. I'd never be part of their club.

Even my mother, who was as close to being a saint as I had experienced in my childhood, regularly used guilt to manipulate us into doing what she wanted. But what else could she do? This was the training of the Church. It was all about being on the in with God, while making others feel as if they were out of favor with the Lord.

As a result, the whole subject of religion landed on me like a bad headache. My training had instilled within me a voice whose purpose, it seemed, was to make me feel badly about myself whenever I was feeling good. Religion could cure you of self-love, if you let it! Sometimes I could clear away my religious beliefs and find comfort in God, but when I saw God through the prism of Catholicism, especially the religion of my relatives, my heart sank. Looking back, I realize that it was no coincidence that when I entered puberty, and felt the stirrings of my womanhood, I started to suffer a litany of strange and unexplainable illnesses. Perhaps my real illness was the emergence of sexuality. When Tom and I got married, I remember experiencing a tremendous sense of relief that it was okay now to have sex because I was married now. No one had ever told me that it was okay to be a woman.

The only way to make being a woman okay was to be compliant and agreeable with men, especially with priests and doctors. Doctors were the secular priests, especially in my house. My grandmother died, my mother said, because my grandmother did not have health insurance. My mother preached that whenever we had the slightest symptom, we should go to the doctor, because we had health insurance. It was a measure of how far my family had come since we had immigrated to America. But it also taught us that doctors were our last hope against grim death. You don't question your doctor—not if you want to live.

Perhaps this explains why, when I started to explore alternative approaches to health, I felt a strange pangs of guilt, as if I was going outside the boundaries of what was approved of by the church. But which church was I thinking about then—the Catholic Church, or the medical one? In my mind, they overlapped so much that it felt like a sin to go against the doctor.

AND THEN ANOTHER CRACK IN THE EDIFICE OF FAITH ○ I fought my doubts about Dr. Gray, and suppressed any questions I might have about the omniscience of doctors. Dr. Gray was my lifeline. If he didn't know the causes of cancer, than who did? He had assured me that, once my leg was removed, my cancer would not spread. How could the cancer jump to another part of my body if it had been confined to my leg, and my leg had been removed? As for the possibility that I might get another cancer, the chances of that were remote, I thought—about as likely as getting hit by lightening twice. Even so, Dr. Gray wanted me to have regular check-ups and MRIs, just to be on the safe side, which I dutifully complied with.

And then somehow the fragile foundation that was my confidence was shaken yet again. An MRI in March 1994 showed that bone cells had turned up in my thyroid gland, located at the front of the neck, between the clavicle bones. None of the doctors I consulted, including Dr. Gray, knew how bone cells could migrate to my thyroid.

Dr. Gray said that about one-quarter of my thyroid would have to be removed. I entered Mercy Hospital in Portland, Oregon, where a surgeon removed half of my thyroid although I had been told prior to surgery that only one quarter should be excised. When I awoke from surgery my doctor informed me that all the bone cells had been eliminated. The remaining half of my thyroid would be sufficient to maintain my metabolism, which meant that I would not need synthetic hormone, my doctor said. There was little solace in his words.

Tom and I insisted on accepting the positive pronouncements of the doctors who told us the bone cells were benign. But we had too much experience at that point not to suspect otherwise.

As if to add insult to injury, I soon suffered a flare-up of colitis, an illness I had not had since high school. Once again, I suffered from terrible cramping, diarrhea, bloody stools, and fever. Immediately, I thought the cause was my change in diet and the increase in whole grains and vegetables. I reduced both and went back to eating more meat, eggs, and dairy products. Eventually, the condition subsided and then disappeared. I concluded that whole grains and vegetables were no good for me.

My body was breaking down, but why? I experienced a fear that bordered on panic and I knew intuitively that my life was out of control. I could not stop the dark process that was underway inside of me. My doctors could keep cutting me up, but sooner or later the cancer would find a place where no surgeon's knife could go.

And then my world was shaken even further. Later that same year, my mother was diagnosed with colon cancer. Doctors removed part of her colon and resected the remaining portions. After she recovered from surgery, no further treatment was recommended. Six months later, the cancer returned in her lung, so she elected to begin chemotherapy, which was followed by radiation treatments. Since she was in Maine and I was in Oregon, I traveled back and forth to see her as much as I could, which wasn't enough for either of us. She was not in imminent danger, her doctors said. At least for the moment, she seemed safe. It turned out to be a long, drawn-out illness and a poor quality of life.

WHERE I COULD BE STRONG AGAIN ○ Behind the experience of a failing body, and life without a leg, lay memories of being strong, graceful, and free. Those memories had been forgotten, or repressed, because after I lost my leg it hurt to recall those memories. But in the middle of a particularly frustrating day, they seemed to coalesce into a compassionate voice that bubbled up from my soul. "Meg, go swimming," that inner voice said. And in an instant, my heart opened and joy ran through my body like healing waters.

We were still members of a pool in Beaverton, though I hadn't gone swimming in a couple of months. The thought of going back thrilled me, but made me nervous and timid, too. I'd be making a very public display of myself in a bathing suit and only one leg. But as I gathered my suit and towels, memories of better times came rushing back to me. My mother used to take my sisters and brother and me to the lake, where we would swim from morning until noon. When we got out of the water, our lips would be blue and our stomachs empty and ravenous. My mother would have lunch waiting for us. We'd be balled up in our towels, while we ate our lunches and laughed at each other. Once we had eaten, we had to wait that magical hour before going back into the water. "It takes an hour to digest your food," my mother would tell us. "You'll get cramps if you go in sooner." And we knew that hour was sacred. But when we had pestered her enough—"Has it been an hour yet? Has it been an hour yet?"—and the hour had passed, we ran back to the water, this time wearing our red woolen sweaters with the gray buttons that my mother had knitted for us. She said they were like old fashion bathing suits—her attempt at making them special. They did keep us warm, though, and that allowed us to stay in the water longer, which was all that mattered anyway.

But now, when I entered the health club that housed the swimming pool, I was deeply apprehensive. How would people react to me? Could I swim as well without my leg and foot? Could I swim at all? I got undressed in the locker room, put on my bathing suit, and went out to the pool on my crutches. As always, there were about a dozen people either in the water, or on the landing surrounding it. Many were older people with whom I was friendly. Recognizing me, they greeted me warmly, but their stares quickly turned puzzled and then frightened as they realized that I was on crutches and that, from below my robe, only one leg emerged. I sat down on a bench, took off my robe and saw the shock on their faces just before I got into the water.

The water was my refuge and I began to swim. My arms turned in long circles and pushed the water back with more power than I realized I had. My leg kicked with all the strength that it once did. My body cut through the water, a wake giving way on either side of me as my handicap seemed to disappear in the water. I felt my body's natural power, coordination, and grace. On land, I was deformed, slow, and clumsy. But in the water, I was strong and faster than most.

Though I would never have admitted it to anyone, I felt a sudden rush of pride rise in my chest. Something inside me was smiling. I'm still a good swimmer, I told myself. I kept swimming. My body moved in rhythm. I turned my head to breathe as my hands, arms, and single leg propelled me through the water, mermaid-like. Gradually, my doubts faded and were replaced by confidence and joy—feelings that I had not experienced since my operation. Swimming was a place from which I could draw strength and courage. In the water, I was almost normal again.

After about an hour, I got out of the pool, got dressed, and returned home. The joy and newfound confidence were still with me when I hobbled into the house.

TO WALK AGAIN • On land, life was more complicated. I dragged my prosthetic leg around like a ball and chain. This thing was supposed to make my life easier, but even when I used it, I still needed crutches to get around. Most of the time the leg was merely clumsy and heavy, but every so often it proved to have a mind of its own. One day, I dropped a plate of food on the floor and fell down while trying to pick it up. When I got up, the leg came loose, causing me to fall again. Infuriated,

I picked up the leg and threw it at the wall, causing an enormous dent in the plasterboard. Oh my God, I thought. I got up and moved a table in front of the dent in the wall and then placed the telephone on top of the table. Maybe people won't see it, I told myself. But sure enough, when Tom got home, he noticed it immediately. When I finished telling him of my frustration, he said, "What are you going to tell people when they ask you about the hole in the wall—that you had a temper tantrum and threw your leg at it?"

I have to have a better prosthetic leg, I told myself. There must be someone in America who knows how to make functional limbs. Not long after I made that frustrated plea to the universe, I found an article in *Redbook* magazine about the prosthetic limb maker who constructed the leg for Edward Kennedy's son, Teddy. Kennedy had lost his leg as a result of cancer. The prosthetist's name was John Sabolich, who in the early 1990s, worked in Oklahoma City. Sabolich headed a team of specialists who made lightweight, natural-looking limbs. When they ran into a problem, they conferred with each other and came up with real solutions. I flew to Oklahoma City and spent three weeks being fitted by John Sabolich's co-worker, Bob Hougland. Hougland had lost his left leg in a railroad accident. This was a man who knew all the struggles and frustrations of prosthetic limbs. Not only could he relate, but he was a real artist and intelligent technician. Bob was good-natured, humorous, and honest. He told me what he could do and what the limitations were. Unlike so many other limb makers with whom I had worked, he made no unrealistic promises, but as is often the case with modest people he gave me the best leg. I spent three weeks in Oklahoma, going through the trial and error of repeated fittings and adjustments for the new leg. But as I put it on and walked a bit, even before Bob Hougland had finished making it, I knew immediately that this was it—a leg that was lightweight, strong, and truly functional. I couldn't wait for him to finish it.

In the meantime, I had to make my way around a city I did not know. Ever since I had lost my leg, I had become apprehensive about traveling on my own and being away from Tom. And with good reason. Walking on the crutches while trying to carrying a small bag on my shoulder could be frustrating. On my trip to visit John Sabolich, I first flew to Dallas and then made a connecting flight to Oklahoma. There was very little time between flights so I had to hurry. I had a carry-on bag that kept falling off my shoulder and tangling itself in my crutches, tripping me.

While I was in Oklahoma for three weeks, I was forced to get around under my own power. I had to figure out what I could carry and what I couldn't; how I could get from one part of the city to another without having to walk too far; where to eat, and what to do when I wasn't being fitted. These things might seem like small challenges, but to a woman who was forced to leave college because of homesickness and panic attacks—and that was on two legs!—these were major accomplishments.

When I finally got home, I had a leg that allowed me to walk again. With it came a sudden rush of hope and life energy. But around the house or near my home, I now could walk around with only my prosthetic leg and a small limp. Soon after, I started walking several blocks and then a couple of miles. And that was freedom.

A PAINFUL DRIFTING APART   ° Things were growing increasingly complicated and distant between Tom and me. Tom had been made head of Research and Development at Nike and now had more than 400 people working under him. It was during those years that Nike went from $800 million a year in sales to $8 billion. Tom and many of his colleagues were at the epicenter of that expansion, which meant that he worked long hours and was frequently gone on trips to Asia, Europe, and throughout the U.S. The distance between us couldn't be measured just in miles, however. We were drifting into our separate worlds, and going in separate directions. Tom was climbing the corporate ladder with the speed of a rocket, it seemed. He was celebrated at work, but suffering at home. My life, on the other hand, was falling like a big rock in deep water, though I didn't realize how fast my life was sinking until much later. Meanwhile, an invisible wall seemed to be growing between Tom and me. And as it grew, we both found it harder to communicate our feelings and feel at peace in each other's company. All we knew was how to take care of the household chores and be good parents. When Tom came home, I asked him how his day had been. "Oh, the usual catastrophes," he'd say. Tom is more ironic than direct. But there was an unmistakable anger creeping into his tone. When he got home, he'd have this aura of anger all around him, as if he wanted me to stay away from him.

"I'm not angry," he'd say when I asked him about the feelings he was giving off. Then he'd go into the living room and watch television. Later in the evening, he'd help the children with their homework, clean up dinner, and, exhausted, we'd go to sleep.

One night, as we lay in bed, I reached over to Tom and held his hand. Tom reacted with anger and pushed my hand away. It was a metaphor for how we interacted during the day. We rolled over on our sides, our backs to each other, and went to sleep—lonelier than ever.

"You practice invulnerability all day long," Tom later recalled, "and then you come home and you're supposed to be sensitive and vulnerable. Looking back, I wish that I had had the tools to be more intimate with Meg. She was working so hard. She wasn't feeling well; she had this heavy leg to drag around with her. Meg couldn't do anything spontaneously. It takes a tremendous effort just for her to get dressed in the morning. And then, of course, she took care of our children, did her shopping, and prepared meals. It took her twice the effort to get through her day than it took for me to get through mine. But a lot of the time I couldn't get to that higher state of awareness where I could operate from that knowing. Instead, I lapsed into behavior that I developed as a kid—you know, self-reliance, never show weaknesses or your needs, always be in control. Isn't that what a man is supposed to be? That was my image of a man. But, yeah, I was angry and hurt, no doubt about it. I just didn't know at whom. I thought I was angry at Meg. The problems seemed to be coming through Meg, so at a superficial level, I let myself believe I was angry at her. But if I really thought about it, I would have realized that I had a lot more compassion for her and a lot more love and respect than anger. We just didn't have the tools to look at our anger and our pain, and express it, and get passed it, so that we could experience the love and respect we had for each other. And then, of course, I never expressed in a very enlightened way, which only made matters worse."

Neither Tom nor I were getting our needs met on any level. We were both struggling to cope as best we could with the unfolding tragedy that was running our lives. Having children helped. Both Cammie and Francis were athletic. Both played soccer and Tom and I went to virtually all their games. And both skied. Cammie was a talented downhill skier and Francis became a freestyle skier. Tom and I focused on the joys and struggles of our children, which occupied most of our days. Tom ran and had his work and travels. Meanwhile, I took care of the children and tried to create as normal a life as I could.

A RETURN TO SIMPLE PLEASURES ○ Once I had the functional leg, my dreams of being one of those exceptional people who can perform all kinds of athletic feats on one leg and a prosthesis started to come back. I had seen video clips of amputees who played basketball and even skied. Basketball's out of the question, I told myself one day, but I bet I can ski.

That winter of 1995, I went home to Maine to visit my family, and as fate would have it, I saw an ad for a skiing resort that offered lessons for amputees. The resort was not far from my parents' home. "Let's do this," I told my sister, Liz. Liz could get lessons for non-handicapped people, while I got the special lessons for amputees. A few days later, Liz, her then-boyfriend, Steve—he later became her husband—and I were on the slopes, learning to ski. I wore this really geeky skiing outfit that included goggles and heavy parka. I remember worrying that I might turn out to be as bad a skier as I looked. The instructor was wonderful, however—very reassuring and full of practical advice. She taught me how to balance on one leg and one ski and how to get up after I fell.

As it turned out, I was a natural. I could ski better on one leg than many people could on two. The only thing I couldn't do very well that first day was stop, which meant that I spent a lot of time using my bottom as a brake. But other than that, I could maneuver down the slopes. Of course, I got the ski bug bad after that. That winter, my son attended a skiing class for children that I later chaperoned. Once the kids were on the slopes, the adults were free to ski. I skied twice a week for the rest of that winter and loved it.

Soon, Tom joined me and got the ski bug, too. Both of our children became champion skiers. But in early 1995, we were all novices, though I had more experience than any of the rest of my family.

That winter, we went to Winterpark, Colorado, where we stood before the great black diamond trails that ran far up into the Rocky Mountains. I felt in awe of the sheer height of the mountain and marveled that anyone could actually ski down such a slope. How could you control your speed and keep from killing yourself? I wondered. That year at Winterpark, I stuck to the beginner and intermediate trails, but the black diamond trail seemed to call to me.

I skied the rest of that season, always wondering what it would be like to ski down that mountain at Winterpark. The following year, we went there again. This time, I skied down that same black diamond trail that, only a year before, had thrilled and terrified me. As I came hurtling down the mountain, other skiers gave me the thumbs-up sign, and shook their fists in celebration, and called out to me. They whooped and hollered in triumph as I sped by. All I could do was smile inside and tell myself that anything is possible—even learning to fly. Later, *McCall's* magazine would do a feature on me for my skiing and because I became a leading fund-raiser for a charity for handicapped people who wanted to learn to ski.

But over the next two years, my headaches and sinus problems became worse. My medications were all increased and I was given new drugs. None had any lasting impact on my pain or sinus trouble, however. I remember being on the ski lift in the winter of 1997 and talking to strangers sitting next to me to distance myself from the realization that I was 60 feet above the ground. I was uncomfortable when the lift stopped; but for the first time in my life, the sheer joy of skiing downhill overcame my fear of heights.

As I spoke to my fellow riders, I took out my medications and popped Klonopin and Hismanal, and then squirted the Becanase cortisone spray up my nose. By that time, taking drugs was second nature to me. I went to my doctors, told them of my symptoms, and they prescribed some new medication that allowed me to live my life. I was blissfully unaware that the drugs were doing nothing to the underlying illness, except to suppress its symptoms. Meanwhile, I was getting more and more ill, though I didn't know just how sick I really was.

5. Getting it wrong, until it's too late.

Hindsight can be devastating in its clarity. As I look back on the years 1996, '97, and '98, I can see clearly that my doctors were not curing any of my health issues. Rather, they were using one medication after another in an effort to silence my symptoms. Unfortunately, they weren't very successful at that either. My doctors were like fire fighters who were trying to put out a forest fire by attacking random patches of the blaze, rather than going to its source. They would attack this symptom or that one, only to have the fire re-emerge in some other part of my body. My doctors saw no connection among my illnesses. My problems were all unrelated conditions, my doctors insisted, and none of them suggested a larger disease process taking place within me.

Meanwhile, there was a bizarre synergy to all of these events. My doctors kept reassuring me that my illnesses were nothing to worry about. Even when I began to manifest terrifying symptoms—symptoms that any ordinary person knows are serious—my doctors acted with the most cavalier attitude, as if a light-hearted approach was enough to make the symptoms less significant.

Contrary to what you might think, I'm not at all bitter about this. I realize today that I was confronting the medical way of thinking, which is fixated on the parts of the body, rather than the whole. From this fragmented tunnel vision that rules medicine, headaches have nothing to do with intestinal disorders, which have nothing to do with swollen lymph nodes or breast cancer.

Today, I see a larger order to it all and embrace the lesson with which I was being confronted. Trust your own judgment, an inner voice was trying to tell me. You know that these drugs are not your answer. You also know that what these well-educated and well-intentioned people are telling you is wrong. For a young woman who hadn't learned as yet to trust herself, that was an important lesson to learn from life. But I was still unwilling to take that step, which meant that I would have to follow the medical course—until its inevitable dead end.

LITTLE SYMPTOMS TURN INTO BIG ONES ○ It was the headaches that kept me returning to my doctor. After its initial effectiveness, the Becanase cortisone spray gradually lost its power against my pain. It also had significant side effects that included bone loss and fatigue. As a replacement, my doctor prescribed Flonase, another cortisone spray that did not have the same side effects as the Becanase. Flonase worked great, at least for several weeks, but like the Becanase its effectiveness slowly tapered off until I had to combine it with over-the-counter medication. This combination of drugs mitigated the pain, but never eliminated it completely.

I was convinced that the headaches came from an allergy to mold, which proliferated in Oregon's perpetual rain and dampness, so I kept a constant army of dehumidifiers humming in the rooms of my house. If enough of these machines were busy, perhaps I could dry out my own little corner of Portland. In the meantime, I visited complementary healers, one of whom suggested that I might have fibroids in my sinuses. Medical tests later proved that theory false. A medical doctor suggested a type of surgery on my sinuses that he thought might give me relief. But I had had enough surgery.

On my own initiative, I went to an ears, nose, and throat specialist who prescribed an antibiotic that would kill any bacteria that might have arisen inside my sinuses and could be causing the headaches. I took the antibiotics for the full six-week cycle. The headaches were unaffected. Instead, I developed colitis.

Three and four times a day I filled the toilet with blood. I also had terrible bouts of cramping, especially in the morning. I realized immediately that the colitis was caused by the antibiotics, which had killed friendly bacteria and disrupted the balance of flora in my intestinal tract. Sometimes the cramps would be so bad that I would be doubled over in pain. At the time, I was trying to eat a healthier diet that included more whole grains, such as brown rice. But when the colitis struck, I stopped the grains because I feared that their high fiber content was irritating my intestines.

I was having trouble with food in general. Within 30 minutes of eating or drinking anything, I had a bowel movement. That meant that I couldn't go anywhere that required more than 30 minutes of driving, or to places like the beach that did not have bathroom facilities nearby.

One day after examining me, my internist looked over my insurance information and said, "Oh, you're not on an HMO plan. You can be referred to a specialist." I went to a gastrointestinal doctor who feared that the colitis might turn into Crohn's disease. The doctor told me that it was an inflammatory disorder of the small intestine. I knew that Crohn's disease was an incurable disorder in which ulcers and sores develop and spread throughout the small intestine. Drugs and surgery are used to slow the spread of the disease, but these are only temporary measures. Eventually, much of the small intestine is removed, until an opening must be made in the abdomen so that waste can be released into a sack that is strapped to the waistline. The prospect that I might develop Crohn's terrified me.

The first drug the doctor prescribed had little effect, but a second, called Asacol, stopped the daily symptoms. Instead, it caused chronic constipation. The intense colitis had lasted for four months. Now, I was chronically constipated, with intermittent bouts of colitis, diarrhea, and bloody stools.

While my doctors were treating my acute symptoms, I would sometimes ask them about a more subtle abnormality—lumps the size of quarters in my breasts and armpits. I had been aware of them since the early 1990s. In 1996, a female physician examined my breasts and said, "Oh, you have fibrocystic breast disease."

"Should I be concerned about that?" I asked her.

"No," she said. "Just continue to have your annual mammograms." I had been doing exactly that. My insurance covered the tests and like most educated, middle class women, I made sure I got a mammogram each year.

The year before, my mammogram was more the subject of humor than it was of concern. I had worn a pair of long metal earrings to my test. When the mammogram pictures were developed, they revealed a long needle sticking right through my breast. The technician was appalled. What was that? she wanted to know. At first I had no idea, but then it hit me: the mammogram had taken a picture of my earring and superimposed it on my breast. Our laughter was full of relief, especially when the mammogram itself revealed no untoward sign of disease. Every mammogram I'd had to that point had been equally reassuring.

By 1998, the lumps that had become more numerous and, the lymph nodes under my arms were the size of large olives. I reported this to my doctors, but they thought nothing of it. "Don't worry about it," one told me. "It's nothing." Very often, their words of reassurance were accompanied by mild dismissal, as if I were an obsessing and ridiculous woman. In a strange sort of way, I appreciated their attitude, because it added to my reassurance. Surely, if there was something to fear, my doctors would not behave in this way, I told myself.

Meanwhile, I kept myself going with my assorted array of pharmaceutical drugs and vitamin supplements. In fact, I hated taking the drugs, but I felt crummy all the time—I had headaches, I was tired and depressed, my intestines suffered, and I had this prosthetic leg that I dragged through the day. Whatever relieved my distress, even a little, was good in my book. Which meant that my three or four cups of coffee each day were like medicine. None of my doctors ever mentioned that coffee might be contributing to, or exacerbating, my headaches, colitis, or the lumps in my breasts or armpits. I didn't think of it either. Or maybe I didn't want to think about it. The emotional and physical lift coffee gave me—not to mention the social support that took place over a hot cup— made coffee an essential part of life.

But the combined effects of my physical problems and the drugs were taking a toll on my mind and heart. I was growing increasingly dull and insensitive to what was going on around me. On top of that, I was often exhausted and depressed, which made me appear distant and detached at times. All of which annoyed Tom endlessly. He wasn't sure what was legitimate and what was self-indulgence. It didn't matter, it seemed. In time, everything about my condition and my perpetual complaints annoyed him, which only drove us further apart. But it wasn't just Tom who felt this way. My doctors, too, subtly communicated to me that I was a hypochondriac.

One day, I was watching my daughter's indoor soccer game and decided to confide in a friend my latent concerns about my fibrocystic breasts. "Meg," my girlfriend said, "I knew a woman who died of inflammatory breast cancer. She had been telling her doctor about her symptoms for a year and she kept on getting the same kinds of assurances that you're getting. I'd be very careful if I were you."

Those words rang a cord, but what could I do? I had no knowledge of what might cause fibrocystic breast disease. And none of my doctors suggested that breast lumps might turn into a more serious disease. Also, I was reassured by my doctors' statement that breast cancer ran in families. No one close to me had ever had the illness, which meant that I shouldn't be too concerned. But beneath all of this logical reasoning, I felt trapped. My doctors were the only source of medical information available to me. Intuitively, I sensed that something was terribly wrong with my body, and my feeling did not evaporate just because my doctors kept telling me the opposite. But who else can you go to for health information if not your doctor?

MORE REASSURING NEWS ○ In the spring of 1998, we were preparing to move from Oregon to Maine, my home state. Tom got a job at Cole-Haan, a high-end shoe company. I was eager to return to Maine for many reasons. It was all too apparent now that my mother was dying. Her cancer had spread from her colon to her lungs and ovaries. She had been receiving chemotherapy and radiation treatment for some time, but the effects were devastating. She had lost an enormous amount of weight and was growing weaker by the day. I needed to be close to her. I also wanted to get out of Oregon. The place was too dark and wet for me. But something even more subtle was urging me to go, a thought born of an inner wisdom that perhaps was aware of all that was happening inside my body. I didn't want to die in Oregon, I said to myself. Whatever the source of my inner knowing, it was soon supported by a strange and unexpected event.

In May, just a month before we moved back to Maine, I was out walking on my artificial leg and using my crutches, which made me use my upper body and pectoral muscles. After my walk, I discovered a large lump that protruded from the top of my right breast. It was the size of a large grape. At its base were a cluster of other grape-like growths. Perhaps my crutches, which supported my body under my arms, had pushed one of my swollen lymph nodes up, I speculated. Whatever it was, it scared me to my core. I immediately called my obstetrician-gynecologist, Dr. Larry Schwarz and showed up at his office just a few hours later in a panic. To my great surprise, Dr. Schwartz was not at all alarmed. "Don't worry," he said. "It's just a swollen lymph node. Women are doing gardening or they're lifting heavy packages. Sometimes these things cause a lymph node to swell and pop out."

Dr. Schwartz was making this pronouncement with the knowledge that for the previous couple of years my pap smears had turned up squamous cells, a red flag for cancer of the cervix. I asked him to refer me to Dr. Harold Lasky who specialized in diseases involving the breast, including breast cancer. I made an appointment with Dr. Lasky who immediately gave me an appointment for a mammogram at his office and a sonogram of both breasts to be done at a nearby hospital. A week later, I was back in his office, reviewing the test results.

According to Dr. Lasky, the test on my right breast, where the lump had emerged, showed no sign of cancer. Then came the "But."

"But if I had any concerns," he told me, "I would be more concerned about your left breast." He then showed me the pictures of my left breast, which were crisscrossed with white, wispy lines, like cirrus clouds in the form of an "S". "This breast is much more suspicious," he said. "But I don't think it's anything to worry about."

His ambiguous statements, in which the words didn't quite match the subtext, continued. Dr. Lasky knew that I was about to move back East. "There are a lot of doctors in Boston who specialize in this and they're very good," he told me. "Maybe you should see someone after you've settled in your new home." I suddenly had the strange feeling that even as he reassured me, he was secretly telling me to get another opinion—after I left town.

Our family moved to Portland, Maine, on June 15, 1998. Before we left Oregon, I had set up an appointment with an oncologist in Maine. Unfortunately, his secretary called me back and said that I could not see the cancer specialist until I was actually diagnosed with cancer. Instead, she recommended I see Dr. Steven McCullough, a kindly, white-haired man in his 60s. We were settled in our temporary home only a couple of weeks before I saw Dr. McCullough. My records had been sent ahead to him and now he looked at the sonograms and mammograms taken by Dr. Lasky and then examined my right breast, paying careful attention to the grape-like growth that still protruded from my breast.

"I'd like to have it removed," I told him when he finished his examination.

"Why," he asked. "For cosmetic reasons or because you're afraid it might be cancerous?"

"Both," I said.

Dr. McCullough went to a metal box of instruments and took out a long needle. He said he would aspirate the lump, draw out some fluid, and have it analyzed. He then tried to insert the needle directly into the growth. The needle had not penetrated much below the growth's surface when a sudden flash of intense pain filled my breast. At that point, the needle could go no farther. Dr. McCullough tried to insert the needle again, this time from a different angle. Again the pain, and again no movement. The lump was like concrete. He put the needle down and then turned to me and smiled.

"Go home and don't worry about it," he said. "It's just a swollen lymph node." His tone was affectionate and patronizing, as if he were talking to a little girl to whom he had just given a lollipop.

You're a nice old man, I thought, *but I'm going to see someone else.*

A MOTHER'S PASSING ○ As pressing as my health problems were, they had to take a back seat to a more immediate crisis. On July 14, 1998, my mother died at her home in Westbrook, Maine. During her last few months of life, the cancer made her a shrunken and withered version of herself. It was horrible watching this woman, who was always so full of life, disintegrate before our eyes. By the end of June, she was choking on her own secretions. I got a suction machine from a local medical supply store and used it to clear her trachea, but sometimes she hacked and wretched until we thought the convulsions alone might kill her. As a distraction, she asked us to put on the television so that she could watch the cooking shows. Her love of food and cooking were with her to the end. The sad irony was that she couldn't eat during the last ten days of her life. The only thing she could get down was popsicles, ginger ale, and Poland Spring water. The intense pain that she suffered required high doses of morphine, but the drug caused hallucinations. She was too weak to tell us what she was experiencing, but she asked that the lights be left on all night long.

Although it was a hot summer, my mother was always cold. She would ask to be covered with blankets in ninety degree weather. We took turns combing her hair, trying to keep her warm, and attending to her other small needs—anything to make her feel loved. There wasn't much anyone could do for her to make her comfortable. My father stayed awake most nights in the event that she needed something, or might pass during the small hours of the morning.

Throughout that last month that I was with her, I would often sit by her side and comb her hair. Outside her window, I could hear the birds chirping. My mother loved birds. Whenever she heard them singing, she would stop the conversation and say, "Listen. The birds are singing." Then she would whistle and try to mimic their song. That often made us laugh. After she listened a while longer, she would look out into the distance and say, "Isn't that beautiful."

My father was at her side, holding her hand, when she finally inhaled her last breath and left this world. The people from the funeral home arrived at the house and put my mother in a plastic bag. Then they placed her body on a gurney and began wheeling her out of the house. Before they got to the front door, my sister Ruth stopped them and unzipped the bag so that my mother's face was exposed. She wouldn't leave the house without her dignity. After the funeral directors left with her body, I went through her small belongings, looking for a necklace with which she might be buried. The only piece that I could find was some cheap costume jewelry, a worthless arrangement of plastic that was a symbol of my mother's selflessness, her generosity toward her family, and her humble life that never sought her own adornment. I held it in my hand, felt its weightlessness, and recalled a stream of memories that broke my heart.

Soon after my mother's death, I saw yet another doctor about my breast. His name was Robert Sylvester, a family practitioner. After examining me and reviewing my records, Dr. Sylvester assured me that it was probably nothing, but if I wanted to pursue the matter further I could see a cancer specialist, Dr. Rebecca Meredith, whose office was in Trinity Hospital in Portland, Maine.

At that point, I was in a confused state. All the doctors I had seen had reassured me that my swollen and lumpy breasts and swollen lymph nodes under my arms were nothing to worry about. Some of these doctors even treated my concerns with condescension, as if I were a sweet little girl who was afraid of the dark. In fact, I was a 41-year-old-woman who, on one hand, accepted their reassuring statements—or at least desperately wanted to—but, on the other, could not deny my unsettling concerns. Deep inside, I knew that something was wrong. Still, Tom and I agreed that the chances of my having breast cancer seemed remote. What were the odds that I would get cancer twice? They were probably as small as the chances of getting hit by lightening twice.

AND THEN THERE WAS THUNDER ○ In early November, I needed a new leg made in Oklahoma City. My residual limb had lost quite a bit of muscle mass and fat, which meant that the artificial leg no longer fit. Before I went, I made an appointment to see Dr. Rebecca Meredith at Trinity Hospital right after Thanksgiving. Then I flew to Oklahoma. Once I was there, I underwent the same tedious process in which a leg was constructed, fitted, and refitted, again and again. The trip was a disaster. I was hoping to stay only two weeks, but we could not get the leg to fit properly and had to stay a fourth week. I was homesick for my family and depressed. What really terrified me was that, on several nights, I was roused from sleep by pain in my right breast. That was a bad sign, I knew. When I took a shower, I would sometimes run my hand over my breast and get this sickening feeling in the pit of my stomach. I could not think about my breast without feeling an immediate flash of fear. If I had let myself dwell on it, I would surely have collapsed into panic. I wanted to run home to the security of Tom and my children, but I couldn't because my leg hadn't been finished yet. So I placed my fear and my homesickness in some corner of my mind until my leg was completed, which happened just before Thanksgiving. The flight home seemed to take forever. But when I got home, I found that my appointment with Dr. Meredith had been pushed back to mid-December.

Nearly three weeks later, I was in Dr. Meredith's office where she examined me and looked over my records. She immediately sent me for a sonogram, which took place inside the hospital. The sonogram technician was a woman, with whom I immediately felt a rapport. I knew the minute she looked at me that she was seeing me and taking me seriously. To do the test, I had to get into a hospital gown and then lie down on a table under the sonogram machine, which she maneuvered to take pictures of my breasts. Within 10 or 15 minutes, she and a male doctor entered the room where I lay. As they did, the doctor switched on the light, came over to me, and introduced himself. It was a routine that I had seen before. In an instant, I knew I had cancer.

"Mrs. Wolff, with your permission, I'm going to do a needle biopsy on your right breast," he said. "Would that be all right with you?"

"Yes," I told him. I felt myself collapsing from within, like a building that had been detonated and was falling into rubble.

"I'm going to start by giving your breast a mild anesthetic so that this procedure isn't painful," he said. I noted the difference in the care and expertise between this doctor and Dr. McCullough.

Once the painkiller had taken effect, he then inserted the needle. The needle penetrated the growth without any resistance. I felt no pain. He withdrew a significant amount of dense tissue and then removed the needle. Despite my anxiety, I was impressed with the care and expertise with which he did everything. The thought crossed my mind: *He's had someone in his family who had to go through this.* Meanwhile, the technician stood nearby, looking on with a certain professional concern.

"What are the chances that this is cancer?" I asked.

"Sometimes we see things like this and they don't turn out to be cancer," the doctor said to me. As he spoke, he looked directly at me with kindness and concern and said, "We won't know until the lab analysis gives us a report." He gave the specimen to the technician.

"Can I get the report before Christmas?" I asked. I remembered working in a hospital when I was an LPN. I knew that things slowed down around the holidays and that reports often get delayed.

"I'll make sure the lab gets this right now," the technician told me. "I'll ask them to work on it right away."

"Thank you," I said, feeling the emotional supports inside me collapse on themselves.

LIGHTENING STRIKES—FOR THE SECOND TIME ○ The wait was interminable, if only because I already knew. Just before Christmas, I was driving my car near our home when I received a call on my cell phone. It was Dr. Meredith.

"Are you sitting down," she said. "If you're not, then sit."

"I'm driving," I replied.

"Pull over and stop the car," she told me. I did as instructed and turned off the car's engine. "Okay, the car's stopped," I said.

"You have stage 3b breast cancer," Dr. Meredith said. "It's invasive and has probably spread to your lymph nodes and perhaps other parts of your body. What you have is serious. You and your husband have to come to my office immediately."

Within an hour, Tom and I were sitting in Dr. Meredith's office. We listened as she told us that the tumor in my breast was very large and it was just the tip of the iceberg. My breast was filled with cancer and numerous lymph nodes might also be involved. The breast would have to be removed immediately. After I had the mastectomy, I would undergo chemotherapy and radiation treatment. That would be followed by tamoxifen therapy. "In the long-term," she said, "we might have to remove the other breast, as well." It, too, was suspicious, she said.

As she spoke, I went into shock. All I could think to say was, "I just don't want to die."

Dr. Meredith looked at me, but said nothing.

That night, Tom and I lay in bed. As usual, I took Klonopin to put me to sleep. Before I went to sleep, I looked over at Tom and noticed that his body was heaving. He had put his face into the pillow to muffle the sound of his crying. I couldn't move. Somehow, the fact that he was crying made me more afraid. I felt myself sinking deeper into the abyss of fear. My heart was closed and my body numb and soon I would be asleep.

6. Surgery, a dangerous seduction, and a tiny light.

Tom and I met Dr. Meredith at her office to discuss what lay ahead for me. Dr. Meredith has wavy brown hair and a no-nonsense, sometimes gruff, New York manner. I had the impression that she was trying to be kind to me, even as she took a certain pride in her direct way of speaking.

She informed me that I had carcinoma "with ductile and lobule features," meaning that the cancer was in both the lobes and ducts of the breast. The tumor that bulged from the top of my breast was the tip of the iceberg; the cancer had infiltrated my entire breast. Very likely, some of my lymph nodes were also filled with cancer. All of this meant that I would undergo a modified radical mastectomy, which included the removal of my entire right breast and many of the lymph nodes under my right armpit. The lymph nodes would be examined by a pathologist to discover if they had been infiltrated by cancer. The surgery would have to be done soon, though at the time she did not mention a date.

Following the operation, I would undergo chemotherapy and radiation, which, very likely, would be followed by tamoxifen therapy, a drug that would interfere with the amount of estrogen in my body. My cancer was supported and even fueled by estrogen. By blocking my body's estrogen levels, it was hoped that the cancer would be deprived of what it needed to survive.

Dr. Meredith spoke with a directness that made me shudder. She wasn't sparing me any of the details, it seemed. Nor was she going to explain, or justify, the treatment protocol that she had prescribed. This is what must be done, she was saying. There's no room for discussion.

Even in my shaken state, I realized that she was not giving me any odds of survival if I underwent the surgery. Nor did she tell me the statistics of women who had the same type of cancer and had survived after treatment. All of this contrasted dramatically with

Dr. Gray's manner. He had explained his thinking at length and justified his medical decisions by telling me that the surgery would save my life. But Dr. Meredith didn't even hint at such a possibility. As she spoke, my mind frantically searched through every sentence, looking for a word or phrase that might give me hope. Every cell in my body seemed to be shouting, *Tell me I'm going to live, right!? Give me something, anything, that I can hold on to.*

Nothing. There wasn't a single word in all that she said that gave me the slightest glimmer of hope. I remained silent, but inside I was a burning engine of fear. "Do you have any women who have had their ovaries removed as a treatment?" I asked her. I had read that some women with breast cancer had even had their ovaries removed to eliminate most of the estrogen from their bodies since it was believed that the removal of the estrogen slowed the growth of the cancer.

"I only had one patient who did that and the results were disastrous," she said.

I asked about breast reconstruction surgery, but Dr. Meredith didn't hold out much hope of that happening, either. "You don't have enough body fat to rebuild your breast," she said. There were other types of breast reconstruction, including the insertion of a silicone implant, but even these probably would not work for me, she told me. Nevertheless, she did give me a name of a surgeon to whom I could talk about such procedures. "There are a lot of people out there that will sell you a cheap suit," she said. "This man won't do that." Immediately, I got the impression that the doctor she was recommending would probably dissuade me from the operation, and Dr. Meredith knew it.

Talk of breast reconstruction was a diversion from all that Dr. Meredith was trying to communicate to me. It was as if we had temporarily entered a fantasy where the appearance and shape of my body still mattered. But the weight of Dr. Meredith's manner brought me back down to earth quickly and her seriousness revealed just how ridiculous the question had been. As if to put a sharper point on all that she was saying, she informed me that the cancer very well may have spread to other parts of my body, including my lymph nodes and left breast. She looked directly into my eyes as she said this, as if to drive the point home. She explained that I would need an oncologist, a doctor who specializes in cancer treatment. I chose Dr. Michael Dowd, who worked at a cancer center in greater Portland. He was highly recommended as one of the best in his field.

I was reeling inside and my mind lost its focus. It was as if I stepped back from the intensity of the moment and my terror-filled body. Suddenly, I noticed the nice wicker furniture in Dr. Meredith's office. I realized that the art on the walls was tasteful and pretty and I wondered if she had chosen it, or if some expensive interior decorator had been hired to dress up the office. I imagined the conversation with the interior designer in which Dr. Meredith described the look she wanted, one that created a certain image for herself. I fantasized about a life in which the ambiance of one's office was important. Dr. Meredith seemed so safe and sure in the place where she was sitting.

"Can you give me any names of women who have undergone the kind of surgery and treatment that I have to go through?" I asked, still searching for any clue that might give me hope.

"There are a couple of women I may be able to refer you to, but I'll have to talk to them first," she said.

The meeting lasted about 30 to 45 minutes and ended without formality.

THE MEDICAL LONG SHOT—AND ITS DARK CONSEQUENCES ○ About a week later, I was in the very posh confines of the cancer center. I had come to meet Dr. Dowd, who would tell me about bone marrow transplant surgery. When Tom and I entered the large foyer, we were immediately greeted by the rich, heavy quilt art that hung from the walls, along with expensive prints and paintings. The building itself was new, large, and modern—a veritable temple dedicated to the ostentatious display of wealth. I was struck by the contrast with Dr. Gray's humble office and furniture, which I always equated with sincerity and dedication. A receptionist greeted us and then directed us down a long, brightly lit corridor to Dr. Dowd's office.

Dr. Dowd was every bit the equal of his building—slick, supremely confident, and overpowering. He examined me thoroughly, paying special attention to the lymph nodes under my right arm. He palpated the skin, searching my underarm with his fingertips.

I felt self-conscious, vulnerable, and a bit off-center as he examined me. "I don't have any swelling in my arm," I offered as a way to break the ice and open the door to perhaps some reason for hope.

"Don't worry, you will," Dr. Dowd said, slamming the door shut on any personal contact. Then he said, "You have cancer in your lymph nodes."

I was shocked to hear that, especially since Dr. Meredith had said that she wouldn't be able to know that for certain until she did the surgery. "How do you know?" I said.

"I can tell," he replied. He then explained that lymph node involvement meant that my illness was much more severe and that conventional treatment had little chance of saving me. Conventional chemotherapy and radiation would kill most of the cancer, but some of those cancer cells would survive the treatment. The remaining cancer cells would multiply and eventually the disease would recur, making it essentially unstoppable once it manifested for the second time. This cancer was going to kill me, he assured me. My only hope, he said, was bone marrow transplant surgery.

Dr. Dowd then proceeded to describe the procedure, which would begin by removing a quantity of the bone marrow stem cells from my hip. This would be done surgically and require general anesthetic. Once some of my bone marrow was removed and preserved, I would be given extremely high doses of chemotherapy that would kill all the cancer in my body. It would also wipe out my bone marrow and immune system. At that point, the bone marrow stem cells would be re-injected into my body. Some of those stem cells would migrate to the bone and regenerate my bone marrow, which in turn would produce immune cells. In a matter of weeks, my immune system would be restored. Meanwhile, the cancer would be destroyed and I would be returned to health.

"There's an 80 percent chance you will be cured," he told me.

I was amazed and confused all at once. Hope, beautiful hope, suddenly ignited in the pit of my stomach and rose into my chest like a flag of victory that was suddenly run up a pole. Eighty percent chance! That's nearly a guarantee! But if that were the case, then why was Dr. Meredith so obviously pessimistic? Why didn't she immediately say that I would require this procedure, and that it very likely would save my life?

Dr. Dowd cut in on my reverie. There were severe side effects, he said. The high doses of chemotherapy drugs could seriously damage my kidneys, lungs, heart, and arteries. I would have to be isolated for weeks while my immune system regenerated. He handed me a sheet of paper with a long list of side effects that normally accompanied the treatment. The chemotherapy drugs could injure the lining of my digestive tract, making swallowing and elimination painful. I could develop infections. Other side effects included severe weight loss or weight gain, diarrhea or constipation, hair loss, joint pain, heart failure, stroke, liver disorders, and death. One-in-five patients died from the treatment itself, the paper informed me. There was no mention of how many die some time after receiving the treatment. I was horrified and Dr. Dowd could see it on my face.

The procedure would cost about $125,000 he said, but he had already had my insurance checked out and he assured me that my provider would cover the costs if I filled out all the necessary paperwork. He looked at me as if from far away. I had the impression that he was sizing me up, wondering perhaps if I was physically strong enough to withstand the treatment.

Stunned, I got up from my chair and told him that I would think about it. The three of us shook hands and Tom and I left in silence. The impression of Dr. Dowd's handshake was still on my palm when we left the building. I was sickened, horrified, and depressed.

THE SURGERY AND ITS AFTERMATH ○ The mastectomy took place on January 25, 1999. My memory of the days that led up to the surgery is mostly lost to me. Even the day of our arrival at the hospital and the preparation for the surgery is vague in my mind. We were in a little cubicle at the hospital. Tom was at my side. I don't remember saying much. All I can recall of that day was my attempts at letting go of my terror and surrendering into God's hands. Such thoughts provided me with some solace. I realized that letting go was the underlying theme of my life now.

The operation was done by Dr. Meredith. There are several types of breast surgeries. The first is a simple lumpectomy, which involves just the removal of the tumor itself. In this case, the breast is left intact, with little change in its shape and size. There is a quadrantectomy, in which a surgeon removes the cancerous tissue and the surrounding margins. After the operation, the breast is somewhat smaller than it was originally; its shape can be altered, as well. A third type is a simple mastectomy in which a surgeon makes an incision under the breast and removes the breast tissue, including the milk ducts and lymph nodes. A modified radical mastectomy requires the surgeon to remove the entire breast, the nipple, and many of the lymph nodes under the armpit. A radical mastectomy is the same procedure, except that much of the muscle beneath the breast is also removed. In all of these cases, the patient undergoes general anesthesia, meaning he or she is put to sleep during the operation.

I underwent a modified radical mastectomy. Dr. Meredith made an elliptically shaped incision, something like the shape of a football, around my breast, beginning at the bottom and extending upward to include the place where the large lump had popped out. Flaps of skin were left intact so that, after the breast tissue was removed, the skin could be sewn together. The incision extended up into the armpit, where 15 lymph nodes were removed. A separate "stab wound" was made on the right side my chest and a #10 Jackson-Pratt drain was placed under my skin so that blood and fluid could flow out of the wound and into a bag that was strapped to my right side. The operation took about two hours to perform.

The next day, I was sent home. We were living temporarily in a small house on the beach. My mother-in-law, Alice, a nurse by profession, came to our house a couple of days later to take care of me. She is that rare combination of strength and caring that was exactly what I needed. The bag at the end of my drain had to be emptied regularly and its contents had to be measured to ensure that I was eliminating appropriate amounts of fluid. Excess loss of blood and fluid could threaten my life. Too little drainage could result in infection. Alice kept track of such details.

In addition, I needed help getting out of bed on my one leg, or getting my prosthetic leg on. I had to be bathed and helped to the toilet. She made food, ran errands, and took care of me and my two children. No matter what I needed, she never flinched, never looked away, and never resisted my requests. Instead, she made the best of things, accepting every request as something that simply had to be done.

I was on painkillers after the surgery and I often drifted in and out of dreamy states of consciousness. Our house was 100 years old, but it was filled with charm. My bedroom window let in the morning light and on sunny days, I watched the pixy dust move peacefully through the shafts of sunlight that came streaming into the room. At night, before I went to sleep, I would lay in the darkness and let go of this world as I fell asleep. I felt myself drifting back and forth between this dimension and the next, like those particles of dust that were suspended in the light. During my excursions, I realized that our house was inhabited by spirits who sometimes surrounded me or passed peacefully through my bedroom. They let me know that they were good spirits, benign and supportive. I wasn't afraid of them, nor of death.

There were ice storms that winter. The wind picked up handfuls of the ocean and threw it hard against the house. Ice formed on the trees and encased all of life. Long stalactites of frozen water hung from the eaves of our house, like spears that warned of death if you approached. Sometimes I pictured our house as a ship and the crucified Jesus as the carved figure at its bow. And then I saw that I was that crucified figure at the front of the ship, battered by the ocean, the wind, the rain, and the spears of ice. The storms would rage, especially at night.

In the past, I often wondered how the birds and small animals survived such nights. Now I was like a wounded bird, huddled in the storm. I was ready to let go if called during the night. Eventually, the storms passed and the sun came out in the morning, and when the conditions were just right, the little bits of dust appeared again in the shafts of light. And the spirits came back and my hold on life got a little stronger.

About a week after the surgery, I had to see Dr. Meredith again in her office. She examined the incision to see how it was healing. She then inserted a long needle into the drain and drew blood and fluid from my chest. She showed me how to squeeze the bag that hung from my chest so that it would create a suction that would draw more blood and fluid from the wound. My chest had to be wrapped tightly with an ace bandage to keep pressure on the tissues. That, too, would keep the wound draining properly.

As I recovered from the surgery, I was forced to face my deformed body. At first, I couldn't bare to look at myself. It was too much for me take in. But one morning, I worked up the courage and examined my chest. A long, thick red line, crossed by dark stitches, ran from near my sternum to my right armpit. The wound seemed to scream with violence, anger, and pain. It didn't belong there. My mind and body rebelled against what I was looking at. All my adult life, I had seen my breast in that place; beautiful, tender, contoured, and natural. That was me. This long dark river of blood and broken tissue was not me. It was unnatural. Somehow, this thing was imposed upon me, against my will. I didn't want this. Something vicious, malevolent, and horrible had taken my breast, just as it had my leg, and replaced it with this hideous wound. Suddenly, I was deeply tired. My remaining leg felt weak and I thought I might faint. I sat down on the toilet and cried.

For weeks after the surgery, I was conscious of my deformed body. Everyone I encountered seemed to present the image of what a human being should look like. People should have two legs; women two breasts. I watched people move effortlessly as they crossed the street, or walk along sidewalks. I noticed mannequins in dress shops and photographs of women in magazines. Soon I realized that I must not watch television or read magazines, because they stressed the importance of women's figures, and insisted that these images were what women should be. I no longer measured up. How could I find myself, or feel good about who I was, if I did not conform to the idealized image of a woman that television and magazines presented?

Sometimes I would indulge in a dark reverie in which I asked myself, which of the two losses — my leg or my breast — was more painful for me to bear? It took me all of a millisecond to know the answer. I would rather have two legs than two breasts — if I had been given a choice. But I never had a chance to choose. All I knew was that my life unfolded in this way. There was one path and I traveled it as best I could. It was a road filled with pain. And now there was no turning back. The loss was permanent. I would never be young and beautiful again. I tried to hide my losses with my clothing and artificial leg. I hid my pain behind the smile I gave to people when they looked at me. Perhaps that was the only beautiful thing I had left. I didn't know for sure. What I did know was that I was hurt, but I wouldn't let myself become bitter. I was alive. I had my children and Tom. And I didn't lose both breasts, I told myself. At least not yet. I was grateful for that.

Tom was as shocked as I was, though at the time neither of us knew how badly we had been hurt. Like me, he retreated from his pain. Both of us looked for refuge inside ourselves. Since he had visited the doctors with me, he knew as well as I did that my life was waning, though neither of us would say that out loud. Years later, Tom would sum up what he felt at the time.

"When the breast cancer was discovered, I felt like our luck had run out," Tom recalled. "'Where do we go from here?' I kept asking myself. When Meg got bone cancer, we had hope, because they could take her leg. We could tell ourselves that the cancer was gone. Then she got the prosthetic leg and we could pretend that things were normal. But when the breast cancer was diagnosed, there were no answers and no place to turn. The doctors were doing all they could do, but it was obvious that they were pessimistic, and we knew it. Every time we talked to a doctor about Meg's chances of surviving, the best they would say was that it was going to be a long, hard battle. Nobody was offering us the least bit of hope that the battle could be won.

"Every night I worried that Meg was about to die, and that's a really hard place to be, especially when you have young children. I did the only thing I could think to do, which was to go to work and try to hold it all together. I kept telling myself that, 'You've got to be strong everywhere — at home and at work.'

"One day, there was an op-ed piece in *The New York Times* written by Anna Quindlen about her sister-in-law, who had just died. It was an incredibly eloquent elegy about this special woman who did all these wonderful things and no one really knew her. I sat there at my desk and read the article and thought that this piece could have been written about Meg. Meg was always making people feel good, even when she wasn't feeling good herself. She did this in big ways and little ways. There were countless times when someone would see her on crutches and ask if she sprained her ankle. And Meg would smile and say, "No, I lost my leg." Right away, the person would become defensive and a little guilty, because they'd be wondering if they had offended her or something. But Meg didn't miss a beat. She'd say, 'Oh no, it's okay. I got sick. But I'm fine now.' She immediately took care of people in that moment, and it endeared people to her because they saw that she didn't have any self-pity or anger. She didn't need to make people feel badly for her. She had it so hard, but in a million different ways, she was always trying to make it easy on others.

"So for me, the Anna Quindlen article was about Meg. I cut it out of the paper and put it away in a safe place. To this day, I still have that article."

SPARED BY AN ANGEL IN A WHITE COAT ◦ Soon after the surgery, Tom and I were back in Dr. Meredith's office so that she could examine the surgical wound and talk about the radiation and chemotherapy. At this meeting, Dr. Meredith told me that five of the 15 lymph nodes she had removed were cancerous, which made my illness even more perilous. Dr. Meredith informed us that when three or more lymph nodes are affected, the disease is regarded as a late-stage cancer. Heroic measures would be needed to save my life. She suggested that I talk to the people at a prestigious cancer institute in Boston.

Tom and I went to the hospital for a second opinion, which was where bone marrow transplant surgery had been invented. We met a young, handsome doctor in his mid-30s, who was dressed in an expensive pin-striped shirt and a yellow bow tie. He had a perfect smile that he flashed throughout our conversation. He described the bone marrow treatment as a possible cure for breast cancer. He said that many women were using it successfully, women with the same type cancer—and the same stage of development—as my own. Without the treatment, these women would be dead today, he said. The comparison to my own condition hung in the air for a few moments and then fell on us like a huge bag of sand. Suddenly, I felt tired, heavy, and afraid. Like Dr. Dowd, this man was supremely confident in himself and in the treatment he was selling. I wanted so desperately to trust him, but I simply couldn't. There was something in his all-too-perfect manner that reminded me of a car salesman. We told him that we'd think about it and get back to him. Suddenly, the physician looked troubled, as if he couldn't believe that I would turn down the offer he had made. We all shook hands and Tom and I left.

I had a gut feeling that bone marrow transplant surgery would kill me and said as much when I saw Dr. Meredith again. She recommended a colleague, at yet another Boston hospital, this time a university medical center, who could give me another opinion on the procedure. Then she said, "Go with your gut, go with your gut, go with your gut."

The following week, Tom and I went to see Dr. Rock, whose office was typical of a teaching hospital—barren of anything superfluous. He had a simple desk with papers stacked high, chairs, book shelves, and little ambiance. He was in his late 50s, I guessed, and exuded thoughtfulness, care, and balance.

He told me that my chemotherapy would be administered at Trinity Hospital. Each treatment would require five hours and would occur every three weeks. The breaks in between were necessary to allow my immune system to recover from the side effects of the chemotherapy. For women with my disease, chemotherapy typically ran for at least six months. However, there was an Italian study, he said, that showed better results if the chemotherapy was administered over a four-month period, followed by two months of radiation treatment, which was itself followed by two more months of chemotherapy. I decided that this would be the best approach for me.

I asked him about the bone marrow transplant therapy, which Dr. Dowd was urging me to undergo.

"I don't recommend it," he said firmly and flatly. "In fact, I urge you to stay away from bone marrow transplant. I'm in on the research and I've been following it closely. So far, the results clearly show that it's not an effective therapy. Those results will be presented later this year at the annual meeting for the American Society of Clinical Oncology. There's nothing in the data to suggest that there's any significant benefit from the treatment, and, as you know, the side effects can be quite severe."

Dr. Rock's frankness took me by surprise. Dr. Dowd and the physician from the other Boston hospital, had just got done telling me that the bone marrow transplant represented my best chance at survival. I already knew that without some form of heroic treatment, I was unlikely to recover. But even as these ideas passed through my head, my intuition was telling me in no uncertain terms that Dr. Rock was speaking the truth. I had enough experience with doctors to spot a medical salesman when I saw one, and Dowd and the cancer institute physician were more entrepreneurs than they were healers. They saw my expensive health insurance card and knew that I could pay for the treatment. Something told me that that's what mattered most to them.

Looking back, I realized now that my intuition was getting stronger as I got closer to death. Yet, my life-long training had taught me to doubt my inner voice. To be sure, Tom and I looked into bone marrow transplant to see for ourselves if there was any value in it. We soon discovered that nobody with breast cancer was getting cured from the treatment. In fact, there were virtually no studies to support the use of these extremely high doses of chemotherapy on women with breast cancer. And the evidence that did exist contradicted those who were selling the procedure, just as Dr. Rock had told us.

We soon learned that breast cancer cells are slow-growing and extremely hardy. Chemotherapy, even at high dosages, cannot kill all of the cancer. On the other hand, it does indeed wipe out the immune system. The problem is, the cancer cells rebound faster than the immune system does. Within a year, the cancer regains its powers and starts growing rapidly—long before the immune system is strong enough to combat the illness. This was the reason up to 70 percent of women with breast cancer that had spread to their lymph nodes died from the illness.

Years later I would learn that chemotherapy makes matters worse by releasing a great abundance of oxidants, highly reactive oxygen molecules that support the life of the cancer. This makes the conditions within the body hospitable to the cancer, but toxic to the immune system, thus further encouraging the life of the disease. Before you know it, the cancer is a monster inside of you, while the immune system is still weakened, compromised, and unable to stand up to the disease. This does not mean that chemotherapy is necessarily the wrong choice. Oftentimes it's necessary. But something must be done concurrently to strengthen and support the immune system's recovery. I did not know this when I started taking chemotherapy, but by some miracle, life would soon lead me to an approach that would do exactly that.

Doctors never tell women anything like this, however. Nor did they explain to women just how slim the odds of recovery were with bone marrow transplant. The extremely high doses of chemotherapy burned the entire digestive tract, from mouth to rectum, making it extremely painful to eat, drink, or eliminate waste. Women became so weakened that they could barely hold up their heads. Meanwhile, they were kept in isolation, which meant that they could not be with their families during their remaining days of life. Many died directly from the treatment, while others were so severely weakened that they died some weeks or months after it—oftentimes before they were able to say good-bye to those they loved. In the end, the treatment did far more harm than good, if any good at all had come from it.

Three years later, *Discovery Magazine* did an expose on bone marrow transplant surgery. The headline of their article stated it all. "Bad Science + Breast Cancer." The expose revealed that doctors were getting rich on the suffering of desperate women. Physicians claimed that there was research to support the treatment, when no such research existed at all. The magazine quoted a leading physician who was among the treatment's greatest practitioners and proponents as saying, "We knew that the treatment was going to kill some people along the way, to be quite honest, but we knew the disease killed everybody." When I read that, I immediately thought about the Hippocratic Oath, whose most basic tenet is, "First, do no harm." In the end, thousands of women underwent the treatment. "All told, the nation spent around $3 billion paying for it, while an estimated 4,000 to 9,000 women died not from their cancer but from the treatment," *Discovery Magazine* reported.

Even before I read the article, my feelings about doctors were changing dramatically. Dr. Gray was the best human being I had encountered in medicine. He was caring, compassionate, and committed to doing his best. But even he was wrong in all too many cases. Far more common were the physicians who spoke to you as if theirs was the final word in any discussion. They acted like oracles, when in fact they were guessing most of the time. And I discovered the hard way that, all too often, their guesses were wrong.

Unfortunately, this was not the worst side of medicine. Many doctors were mere entrepreneurs, business people, who seized upon unsupported treatments purely for monetary gain. Some of these practices offered nothing more than terrible pain and premature death. That is especially common in the fight against cancer, where experimental treatments, with little therapeutic value, are offered every day to desperate people.

At that point, I had only a small inkling of the lesson that I was trying to learn, which was to trust myself and my own judgment. I didn't realize it at the time, but I had known at every critical juncture what was happening inside my body, and what the best form of treatment was for me. Oftentimes, I knew more about my own health than the doctors who were examining me. Even as they were telling me that my bone cancer would not recur, I felt it growing inside of me. Even as they patted me on the head and told me to stop worrying, I knew I was ill. And even as they told me that I needed bone marrow transplant surgery, something inside of me said no. What I didn't realize then was that this inner knowing could be trusted to guide me out of the storm.

CHEMOTHERAPY BEGINS ○ In late February, I got my first dose of chemotherapy. The regimen was made of three different drugs, referred to as 5fu, cytotoxin, and adryamicin. A port was installed into my chest that allowed the drugs to drip directly into my aorta, the main trunk of the arterial tree that rises out of the left side of the heart. The chemotherapy was administered in a large room full of people who were also battling cancer. Tom drove me to the hospital and I took my place along side my fellow patients. Each of us was attached to a tube that ran to an IV bag, which was suspended from an IV stand. We sat together, commiserated, and got to know each other, as the drug dripped silently into our bodies.

That night, when I got home, I barely made it to the toilet before I began throwing up. I wretched so violently and for so long that I thought my stomach would launch itself into the toilet. After it was over, I was exhausted. I struggled to get into bed but soon found that I couldn't sleep. The drugs turned my nerves on edge and made my body tense and restless. The next day, I could not get out of bed. My mother-in-law came to stay with me. With her help, I finally managed to make it to the bathroom. I sat on the toilet and absent-mindedly ran my hand through my hair, causing great clumps to come falling out.

A few days later, my mother-in-law took me out to buy a wig. When I got home, I took the wig out of the bag and placed it on the kitchen table. My son, Francis, then 12, came into the room and asked me why I bought a wig. "Your hair looks okay, mom," he said. "You don't need a wig." Unconsciously, I reached up and touched my hair, causing a large clump to fall out. I looked down at Francis and saw that he was in a state of shock. His eyes went out of focus and he stared at me in disbelief. I sat down beside him and said, "It's okay, Francis. I'm fine. I'm taking this medicine for a little while and it's causing my hair to fall out. My hair will grow back. You'll see."

"Okay, mom," he said. With that, he ran off to his room.

In the weeks that followed, I sunk ever more deeply into sickness and fatigue. I was already thin, but somehow I managed to lose more weight. My cheeks became hollowed out gourds, my skin turned sallow, my eyes widened and bulged. My hair disappeared. Finally, I looked like a victim of the holocaust that is cancer.

At one of my regular visits to Dr. Meredith, I asked if she could recommend a physician who practiced alternative medicine. No, she said, but she did know a naturopath by the name of Devra Krasner. Within a few days, I was in her office. During our visit, I asked her if she knew of any doctor who administered vitamin C therapy. I had read Norman Cousin's book, *Anatomy of an Illness*, in which Cousins describes his use of vitamin C and laughter to overcome a life-threatening illness.

"Yes," Devra Krasner told me. "Dr. Joseph Ping is a physician who specialized in the treatment of chemical sensitivity. He provides his patients with high-doses of vitamin C therapy."

Soon, my visit with Devra Krasner was over. I thanked her for her help and then started for the door, but before I left, Devra called after me. I turned toward her.

"You know," she said, "some women with breast cancer have been helped by the macrobiotic diet."

Suddenly a light went on inside of me. My heart momentarily opened. That's right I said, as if remembering something that had been told to me in a dream, or perhaps in another lifetime. That's what I'm going to do.

7. *Dying by the hard path, living by the soft.*

It was early March 1999 and small hints of spring were starting to appear. During the fall and winter months, the light had been thin and watery. There had been deep snow on the ground and darkness in the forests. But now, spring was rising as if from the earth beneath my feet. There was a yellow light moving in the trees and daylight was pushing back the night.

I was undergoing chemotherapy treatment every three weeks. My treatments were scheduled to continue until June, at which time I would undergo three months of radiation therapy, followed by another two months of chemotherapy.

The chemotherapy felt like death itself. I would sit under the chemo drip for five hours and then Tom would drive me home. The treatment left me dizzy and disoriented at first, but by the time I got home, the nausea would kick in and I would suddenly become violently ill. I barely made it to the toilet after each treatment. I did not believe it was possible to throw up for so long, or so often, especially when there was nothing left in my stomach but digestive juices. After one of the early treatments, I telephoned my oncologist and in a low, hoarse voice that was barely audible, I asked, "What can I take for the nausea?" He prescribed a medication, which had little effect. I still became violently ill.

Every cell in my body was sick. It didn't matter how much I vomited; there was no relief from the nausea, which was not what I expected. In the past, throwing up always relieved the nausea. But with chemotherapy, there was no such relief. Why doesn't the nausea pass? I asked myself, half dead from sickness and exhaustion. Because the problem isn't in your stomach, I realized. You're being poisoned through your veins. It's in your blood. It's in every cell in your body. The hacking and convulsions were so bad at times that I knew I was just one step away from death. I held on for dear life.

When the vomiting finally relented, I would take off my leg and my wig and lie in bed, fragile, wounded, and utterly spent. On good days, I would fall into a fitful sleep, only to wake up every couple of hours, my body clenched tight with tension, joint pain, and nausea. Usually, I spent the first few days after a chemo treatment in bed, too tired to get up, even to make it to the toilet. I bought a commode and crawled over to it throughout the day. The portable toilet came to symbolize my disease and all the suffering that was associated with it. I hated the sight of it.

Once on the chemo, I immediately went into menopause—I was only 41 years old. I also lost weight. I was already fairly thin, but what little muscle and excess I had seemed to melt away from my body. My clothes were loose now, which made me feel—and appear—even thinner than I was. Even worse, my prosthetic leg no longer fit tightly on my residual limb. I was constantly attempting to adjust it, but without much success. I would have to have another leg made, I realized, but I could not travel to Oklahoma—or anywhere else, for that matter. As the leg got looser, it felt even heavier and more artificial.

Meanwhile, dark hollows appeared in my cheeks and my eyes bulged just a little. The outline of my skull began to emerge in stark relief from beneath my skin. One look at me and people knew.

The dark truth at the center of all my suffering was that no one had even suggested that the drugs were going to save my life. Chemotherapy was simply the accepted course of treatment for breast cancer. My doctors made it clear to me, however, that there were no promises and, in all likelihood, the cancer would kill me. There was never a shred of hope offered, except from the doctors who were pushing the bone marrow transplant.

Among the odd consequences of the chemotherapy was that my mind had become even duller. I became forgetful and often lost contact with the present, as if I were moving in a dream world. The chemotherapy had thrown my body and mind into a state of shock. Some days were better than others. At times I would be clear and present, but then I would inexplicably drift away and lose track of what was happening around me. In truth, something else was guiding me now. My mind had been turned off, but some other mysterious power, perhaps communicating to me through my intuition, was urging me to walk through the door that had been offered.

That door, and my only hope, was macrobiotics. Even in my weakened condition, I felt a sense of hope and purpose when I considered the macrobiotic diet. And every cell in my body seemed to push me to find out more.

Once the chemo sickness had passed, I gathered myself and went to the Whole Grocer store in Portland, where I bought some whole grains, vegetables, and some natural snacks. I also bought two cookbooks, one by Aveline Kushi, entitled *Introducing Macrobiotic Cooking*, and another by Christina Pirello, entitled *Christina Cooks*. When I got home, I started reading the books and then I cooked some of the brown rice and vegetables. Afterwards, I ate hummus on rice cakes. The food was almost tasteless, but somehow I knew that this was the way. I don't even know why or how I knew. The food was simple, yet there was a power in that simplicity. It was as if all of nature had been distilled into every single grain of rice, and every leaf of kale. I was sure that if I knew how to prepare these foods, I could make them tasty and enjoyable, even without sauces or oils, which I often used to flavor the rice and vegetables I had made in the past. What I needed, I realized, were cooking classes. I also needed instruction in the macrobiotic diet.

A few days later, I returned to the Whole Grocer and looked on the store's bulletin board for anyone advertising macrobiotic cooking classes in Portland. There was a single name, Lisa Silverman, who offered macrobiotic cooking classes at The Five Seasons Cooking School. I wrote down the telephone number, drove home, and made an appointment to see Lisa Silverman.

I drove to Lisa's house in downtown Portland. We sat in her kitchen and talked about her classes and I told her that I wanted to eat macrobiotically to help me recover. I was ill and uncomfortable in my body, having just completed another round of chemotherapy. My wig was hot and I felt myself sweating under its artificial surface. All of this distracted me. In addition, chemotherapy left my mind feeling foggy and a bit lost.

Lisa, meanwhile, seemed distracted. Years later, she would tell me that she was upset and intimidated at how terrible I looked. Advanced cancer frightened her, as it does many people. At the time, I didn't realize how horrible I really looked, or how much my presence terrified people. Perhaps I was better off not knowing. Still, I was aware that we weren't making a connection, but I am not the type who judges people on first impressions. If I don't connect to someone on the first encounter, I tell myself that I'll get to know the person and learn to like her or him. Relationships need time and understanding, and I was more than willing to give this relationship all it needed. Lisa held cooking classes one evening a week. She also prepared macrobiotic meals for take-out three times a week. I was thrilled. Not only would I learn to cook, but I could eat Lisa's meals three days a week! I left Lisa's house full of hope.

The drive home, however, proved nearly too much for me. The high I felt after meeting Lisa very quickly consumed all my available energy. My body seemed to collapse into a state of utter exhaustion. I struggled to hold the wheel and concentrate on the road. I realized that just listening to people made me tired. I barely got home and made it to my bedroom, where I fell on the bed and into a deep sleep.

A COMMUNITY OF THE DYING ○ Every three weeks, Tom and I got into the car and drove to Trinity Hospital, where I received another five hours worth of chemo. Very often, Tom would bring a book or work from the office and sit with me. I would read or talk to the dozen-or-so people who sat beside me in the medium-size room where chemotherapy was administered. We would tell each other about how we were coping with the side effects of the chemotherapy, or what we were doing to keep our spirits up. One man, who was in his late-60s, was dying from kidney cancer. He had been divorced and was now living alone. Like most of us, he couldn't sleep most nights, even though he was utterly exhausted. He would lie in bed, look out the window or up at the ceiling, and think about his life. It was heart-breaking for those of us who listened to him.

"Don't feel sorry for me," the old man said to me one day. "I feel sorry for you. You're young. I've lived my life."

The thought of having to go through all of this alone made me shudder. Tom and I had been through a lot of hard times, especially since I had become ill, but there he was, sitting next to me, reading his book, and waiting to take me home.

Our little chemotherapy group worked hard to keep our spirits up. A cute little man named Saul brought in his stamp collection that he had accumulated during most of his life. He showed us many valuable stamps that he had obtained over the years and the story that was attached to each stamp. Another man, named Robert, concluded his chemotherapy protocol and we threw him a party, complete with cake and party favors. He was gay and brought in his partner for everyone to meet. We all celebrated his graduation from chemotherapy as if he would live forever. But before the party was over, the doctors wheeled an elderly patient on a stretcher and inserted the chemo drip into the patient's arm. The person on the stretcher was unconscious and we couldn't make out if it was a man or a woman. All we knew was that he or she was just about dead, and the chemotherapy would only hasten it. From time to time, each of us would cast furtive glances at the stretcher and then quickly look away. Is that me a few months from now? I wondered. No, I told myself. I have a way out of this.

I had macrobiotics, which I increasingly saw as the light at the end of this long and dark tunnel. Only this diet and way of life offered me the slightest hope and inspiration. All else was darkness, despair, and pain.

After every chemotherapy treatment, I visited Dr. Joseph Ping, a Portland osteopath who specialized in treating people with chemical sensitivity. Dr. Ping was in his mid-40s. Unlike so many other doctors, Dr. Ping had an inquisitive nature and an open, supportive manner. At my initial visit with him, he questioned me closely about possible exposure to chemical toxins in my youth, or some other potential causes of my cancer. He also wanted to know about macrobiotics and how it might be affecting my health. Dr. Ping gave me between 25,000 and 40,000 international units of vitamin C, which he administered by placing a hypodermic needle directly into my chemotherapy port.

The vitamin C did not noticeably change my condition. However, it did provide a significant dose of antioxidants, which would boost my immune system, especially after it was ravaged by the chemotherapy. Chemotherapy drugs kill both cancer and immune cells, which means that both are weakened, just as the overall body is. Unfortunately, the chemo also releases an abundance of oxygen free radicals, or oxidants, into the system, which support the life of the cancer while depressing the strength of the immune system. Yes, the chemotherapy may be necessary to weaken the disease, but medicine provides nothing to support the strength of the immune system, which is the patient's only real defense against the illness. In the wake of the chemotherapy, the conditions actually support the restoration of the cancer, which increases the odds of recurrence. Once the cancer recurs, it is nearly impossible to stop it, which is why recurrence is associated with such high death rates. Vitamin C therapy introduces an abundance of antioxidants that neutralize many of the free radicals, and supports the recovery of the immune system. Though this was just a small supportive step, I felt that at least I was doing something to help my body recover.

Vitamin C was not my answer, I realized, but it might support the answer, which was macrobiotics.

WHERE THERE IS HOPE... ○ Anywhere from eight to 20 people attended Lisa's classes each week and everyone got to know each other. It was a little community, one full of hope and inspiration. People came from all over the Portland area to study cooking and the macrobiotic philosophy with Lisa. No one in the group was suffering from cancer, but many of them knew someone who had cured themselves of the disease with the macrobiotic diet. People told me about a middle-aged acupuncturist from Yarmouth, Maine, who had childhood leukemia and used the macrobiotic diet to get well. He had undergone chemotherapy, but was not expected to survive. His mother adopted macrobiotics and prepared all of his foods with an almost religious conviction. When he did survive, his doctors told him that he would never have children, but today he is married and is the father of a twelve-year-old daughter.

There was a man in the class who knew a woman, Nancy Barstow, of Maine, who cured herself of breast cancer with macrobiotics. I later read about her in an article published in *East West Journal*. Eventually, Nancy and I would meet and become friends. People in the class told me about many other people who were at least as bad off as I was and who got well.

Lisa's classes were a wonderful mix of cooking instruction, common sense, and macrobiotic philosophy. Macrobiotics, Lisa taught us, is based on the ancient Chinese philosophy of yin and yang, the two forces that the Chinese believed shaped all phenomena. Macrobiotics combined the science of nutrition with the use of yin and yang to create a healing diet, and indeed a healing system.

Yin, Lisa said, is the force that causes things to expand and rise, yang causes things to contract and descend. Lisa was always very expressive and talked with her hands to accentuate her points. As she explained yin and yang, she raised her arms in the air and opened them wide to illustrate expansive and rising energy, and then slowly closed them and brought them down over her table to demonstrate contraction and descent. I struggled to comprehend all that Lisa was saying. This was important to me and I had to understand it, I told myself.

Every food has either a yin or yang effect on us, Lisa instructed. Yin foods, such as fruit, fruit juice, sugar, alcohol, and certain drugs (marijuana, for example, and many pharmaceuticals) have a yin, or expansive effect. They cause relaxation, diffusion of energy, and ultimately lethargy and reduced movement. In the body, yin foods cause organs to expand and relax. With excess consumption of yin foods, organs become expanded, tired, and weak. They accumulate waste products, become deformed, and ultimately fall victim to illness. Excess consumption of alcohol, for example, causes the liver to become swollen, fatty, and ultimately so packed with free radicals and waste products that it becomes scarred and hardened. Yin foods typically affect the upper part of the body, at the diaphragm and above, including the heart, pancreas, spleen, liver, upper part of the lungs, neck, head, and brain.

Yang foods, such as salt, beef, eggs, and hard cheeses, cause organs to become excessively contracted, sclerotic, and stagnant. They make arteries hard, tight, and eventually closed, thus depriving blood flow to the heart and other organs. They do the same to muscles and organs, thus leading to increasing levels of waste accumulation and stagnation. Yang foods tend to affect the heart and organs below the heart, such as the lower part of the lungs, digestive tract, large intestine, and reproduction. Excess consumption of animal foods are associated with high rates of heart disease and many forms of cancers, for example.

Yin and yang are constantly attracting each other to create balance. People who eat a lot of yang foods, such as beef and eggs, suffer from their contracting effects on the body and therefore are attracted to yin foods, such as sugar or alcohol, to create a more balanced or relaxed condition. For example, bartenders put salty peanuts (yang) on the bar in order to promote drinking (yin). After a hard day of stressful work (yang), people want dessert, sugar, or alcohol (all yin) to help them relax.

All foods can be categorized as having yin or yang effects. However, many foods have far more gentle expansive or contracting influences, while some are more extreme. The more extreme the food, the more extreme the side effects. Sugar and apple juice, for example, are both considered yin, but sugar is far more expansive and weakening than apple juice. Fish and beef are both yang, but beef has a much more contracting and stagnating effect on the body than fish.

Whole grains are considered slightly yang, but not nearly as yang as fish, or foods that are more contracting than fish, such as chicken, eggs, and beef—three foods that are increasingly more yang. Beans are considered less yang than grains. Vegetables, in general, are considered yin. Root vegetables are the most yang of the vegetables. More expansive are the round vegetables (such as onions, cabbage, and squash), and even more yin are the leafies (such as mustard greens, kale, and collards). Fruit is more yin than vegetables and fruit juice more yin than fruit. In general, the more processed a food is, the more yin it is. The foods most of our children are eating—soda pop, sugary snacks, cookies, pastries, and candy—are all extremely yin. They are packed with non-nutritional, or empty, calories. As yin foods, these cause the body to expand, thus resulting in overweight and obesity.

Health is the result of balance within the body. A balanced condition results in greater range of motion within the body—that is to say, less extreme contraction or less extreme expansion. Such a condition is associated with greater blood and lymph circulation, for example. Balance also results in a more relaxed body, greater amounts of energy, deeper sleep, and a stronger immune function. As I would later learn, the macrobiotic diet is packed with immune-boosting and cancer-fighting chemicals. (See Part II)

Macrobiotics recommends eating foods that fall more in the center of the yin-yang-spectrum. That means that the core diet is composed chiefly of whole grains, fresh vegetables, beans, sea vegetables, and fruit, with small amounts of fish (on the yang side) and minimally processed sweeteners, such as rice syrup and barley malt (on the yin side). Such a diet will result in a balance between yin and yang, and a balanced condition, the result of which is health.

Soon after I started attending Lisa's classes, I came to understand that my breast cancer was caused largely by an excess of yin foods, including ice cream, soft cheeses, milk, processed foods, coffee, and sugar. In order to heal, I had to eliminate these foods from my diet, along with all extremely yang foods, such as excess amounts of salt, beef, chicken, eggs, and hard cheeses. My diet had to be balanced and, what macrobiotic people called "clean," meaning free of oily foods and any dairy products, which collectively block blood flow to organs and promote disease, especially cancer.

Even though no one in Lisa's class had breast cancer, most of those who attended were attempting to eat macrobiotically to overcome some form of chronic illness. And most of them were experiencing symptoms of recovery. Many reported greatly improved energy levels. Others experienced relief from chronic symptoms that had plagued them for years. All around me, people were getting well. Needless to say, this had a profoundly positive effect on me. And it came in an atmosphere in which we were learning the most remarkable insights into nature, the human condition, and life itself.

Sometimes Lisa invited macrobiotic teachers to lecture on diet and health. These teachers showed us how a diet rich in animal foods, fat, processed oils and flours, artificial ingredients and pesticides, poisoned the human body and gave rise to all the common illnesses, including heart disease, cancer, high blood pressure, arthritis, Parkinson's and Alzheimer's disease. They were criticizing the very foundation of American culture, our daily food. The standard American diet was the hidden cause of widespread disease and death. That meant that these foods were also the foundation for the medical and pharmaceutical industries, which profited from all the sickness from which we suffered. Even more amazing, Lisa was showing us how we could use simple, natural foods to recover our health. That, of itself, was a miracle, especially for someone like me, who, for the first time, was experiencing real hope. But Lisa went on to show that yin and yang were the basis for a new view of life and a kind of spiritual transformation. I had no idea what that might mean and to be perfectly honest, I didn't care. All I wanted was to get well. My concerns were about life and death. But all of what Lisa said, even the things that didn't entirely make sense to me at the time, were immensely inspiring. It was all new and fresh to me. I was learning something that was altogether foreign, yet immensely personal and helpful. It was as if I had been led to this living room, and to this little group of people, who had been given insights into illness and health that had been hidden from the masses. I felt privileged to be here and overwhelmed with gratitude.

Our little group bonded on so many different levels. Every week we greeted each other and got the latest update on how we doing on the macrobiotic diet, and what, if any, changes were occurring in our condition. All of us knew that we were part of something special—that no matter what our circumstances, this was an important time in our lives.

But there was a shadow, of course. When we left Lisa's living room, we realized just how alone we really were. Three times a week, I would drive to Lisa's house and buy a meal for myself. Sometimes I would be so tired from driving that I had trouble making it home. Instead, I drove down to Casco Bay in Portland and parked near the water on the Eastern Promonade. I turned off the engine, opened the containers of food, and ate Lisa's meal by myself, as I looked out over the cold, lonely water. I often thought about the book by Jean Kohler, the Ball State professor who had cured himself of pancreatic cancer with macrobiotics. In his book, Kohler wrote about how isolating macrobiotics had been for him. He lamented the fact that he could no longer eat in restaurants with friends, or attend social functions, because he couldn't eat the foods everyone else ate. I was lonely, too.

Tom and the children were not eating macrobiotics—they ate whole grains and vegetables, but they also ate dairy products, eggs, and, occasionally, even red meat. And, in the early going, none of them understood my connection to this diet and lifestyle. Tom supported me completely, but he saw macrobiotics as my way of helping myself, and not as something that might help him, too. Now I knew the isolation Kohler wrote about.

In Korea and Japan, my diet and behavior would have been perfectly normal. To begin with, the Asians ate these foods and understood the importance of diet in self-care. One didn't just submit to the doctor for treatment. Koreans and Japanese recognized the need to take responsibility for their health. Many of them did what they could to help themselves. But in the U.S., everything that I was doing was completely foreign and, for many, considered ludicrous. How could diet play a role in the treatment of cancer, the most feared disease of our time? My behavior would have been the basis for ridicule among many Americans—certainly among many doctors. Even many of my relatives and in-laws saw macrobiotics as a desperate, and futile, attempt to survive.

Fortunately, Tom understood what I was doing. He knew that the odds were against my survival, and that anything I did to help myself was not only positive, but essential. This was my only hope, and I held on to it like life itself.

PREPARE YOUR SOUL, HE TOLD ME ○ By late May, my first round of chemotherapy treatments was close to being finished. Just before they ended, and right before I began my radiation treatment, I met with the radiologist, Dr. Allen, who would oversee my treatment. We met just a few days after I had undergone yet another round of chemotherapy. When I showed up at his office, I was deathly ill. Dr. Allen was a religious man with a compassionate nature. He took a long look at me—the weight loss, the gray skin, the slightly bulging eyes, and the weakened state. Meanwhile, I looked back at him and saw his fear and concern.

"How are you feeling?" he asked me.

"Oh, I'm okay," I said with a little smile. I knew that he was an empathetic man and I didn't want to put my troubles on him.

"You're really having a rough time," he told me.

"Yeah," I said, "but I'm doing all right. Don't worry. I'm going to make it," I said.

Dr. Allen took a long pause, as if considering what he was about to say. "Are you religious?" he asked me.

"No, not really," I said.

"You should prepare your soul," he said in a quiet voice. His words fairly shocked me. "You need to start thinking about preparing your soul for God." He kept speaking, but I no longer heard a word he was saying. He was telling me that I had to face the fact that I was going to die, but even as I heard his words, I was actively screening their impact from my heart. Maybe this was one of those moments when I was saved by chemo brain—the tendency of my mind to shut itself off. I drifted into some fog-bound state and waited for him to finish, all the while keeping a pleasant little smile on my face. Perhaps some part of my mind was telling Dr. Allen, "I'm not hearing you."

He meant well, but he didn't have to tell me that I was dying. Besides, the condition of my soul was my business. Still, as much as I tried to keep my death from my mind, I was compelled on a regular basis to consider what my family would do without me. Whenever I thought about my children growing up alone, my heart broke and I collapsed in tears. I tried not to think of them alone. But sometimes I couldn't help it, especially when they seemed so vulnerable, such as when they were playing soccer. We tried to do all the normal things that families did, and soccer was a big part of my children's lives. They'd be running for the ball, completely engrossed in their game, and I'd suddenly be worried about them being motherless. And that would tumble into other thoughts, such as where would I be when they were 16 years old? Without even being aware of it, I would fantasize about buying my son and daughter presents for their sixteenth birthdays. Francis was 13 at the time, and Cammie only 9. I pictured their parties, the house filled with their friends, and them receiving gifts from me, though I'd be long gone by then. It was too much for me to bear.

I didn't want the children and Tom to be alone after I died. So I began to consider other women as potential wives for Tom and mothers for my children. Tom needed to marry again, I decided, but he had to make the right choice. I regularly evaluated my friends as possible mates for Tom. Finally I decided on Kathy, a friend and a member of my book club. Kathy was a beautiful woman, just a couple of years younger than I, with two children of her own and in the process of a divorce. She was soft, friendly, and kind to her children. Tom and Kathy would make a good couple. I decided not to say anything to Kathy and Tom just yet, but when I was down to my last days, I would tell Tom that she was my choice.

THE COLD LIGHT OF RADIATION THERAPY ○ In June, I started my radiation treatments. Finally, I got a break from the chemotherapy. It was like being released from torture. The radiation took place in the basement of General Hospital in Maine, or should I say the dungeon. It was everything that you might expect—dark, cold, the ceiling lined with exposed plumbing. I waited for awhile in the cold, dark basement. All around me were people who were also waiting for radiation treatment. Some of them had already been hospitalized. These people were on wheel chairs, or on stretchers. They were dressed in their hospital Johnny's and nothing else. Most of their bodies were naked—their backs were exposed, as were their bottoms and legs. I was fully dressed, but I was cold. These people must have been freezing. Why were they only in hospital gowns? I asked myself. Couldn't they at least come down here in pajamas and robes? Not only were they cold and uncomfortable, but their dignity was stripped from them.

All too often, doctors don't care about people's dignity. In the radiation ward, patients were little more than bodies to the technicians and doctors. Line them up for radiation, zap them here and there, and then wheel them back to their rooms was the mentality that governed this place. The doctors didn't care about the human part of medicine, the part that embraces the vulnerability of people, their fears, and their tenderness. Doctors had rejected the heart. They were only interested in control, and if you were fully dressed and had your dignity intact, you were a little more difficult to control than someone who was naked and cold.

Finally, I was called into the radiology room. A technician arranged for me to stand in a particular place while he aimed the beam directly at the area of my right breast. A second technician stood behind a wall. He would turn on the machine when his colleague gave the signal. I tried to make a joke and engage the technician in a little light conversation. He turned away from me without acknowledging that I had said anything. The rest of the radiotherapy was done in silence, except when the technician commanded that I turn my body so that the beam might get a better shot at me.

The whole experience was dehumanizing and painful. Yes, it was a relief to be free of the chemotherapy, if only for a few months, but coming here presented another kind of suffering. Somehow, I was less human to these men and women. They didn't understand how important it was to me to be treated with just a little kindness and a little respect. That alone would have lifted my spirits. They didn't want to see me. All they wanted to do was zap me with the radiation and get me out of there.

What so many doctors and technicians fail to realize is that cancer isn't just a disease of the body. It's an attack on the mind and spirit, as well. People with cancer are constantly struggling to maintain their spirits and feel good about themselves. This is pretty simple stuff, and you would think that doctors who specialize in the treatment of cancer would know such things intimately. But that's not the case at all. Many doctors seem not to care how patients feel, which means that people with cancer not only have to battle the disease, but also the cold indifference from doctors. Perhaps it's not that doctors don't care, but rather they are not trained to handle the emotions associated with caring for very ill people. I realized that many medical professionals have little understanding of human nature, and even less of healing.

I left the radiology lab that day telling myself I was still alive—neither the cancer, nor the treatment had killed me yet.

TURNING MORE AND MORE TOWARD THE ALTERNATIVES ○ I was scheduled to undergo radiation treatment five days a week, but the radiation machine kept breaking down on Fridays—a curious coincidence, to say the least—which meant that I was irradiated only four days each week. The four-day cycle worked in my favor, as it turned out, because it gave my skin three days to heal. Later I met a woman who was undergoing the standard five-day protocol. Her skin was fair and sensitive. She told me that the radiation had caused third degree burns and by the third day of treatment her skin was weeping. So I counted my blessings, and thanked God for disabling the machine (or giving the technicians something better to do) every Friday.

Three days a week, I received acupuncture treatments from Fern Tsao, a Chinese doctor from Taiwan who had been in the U.S. 30 years. Fern was barely five feet tall and thin as a needle. Her soft features, warm smile, and lots of vitality give her an ageless quality, though she is in her early 60s. Fern embodies so much of what is magical, mysterious, and wise in the Chinese character. She is extremely sensitive, even delicate, and at the same time strong and loving. Her bearing is full of wisdom and intuitive perception. There is something ancient about her and at the same time incredibly youthful and almost childlike. Fern became my Chinese mother, treating me with her immense sensitivity and kindness.

Every time I entered her office, I felt as if I were stepping into another world. Fern would have me lie down on her acupuncture table as soft, Chinese music played in the background. I would fall into a deeply relaxed state, thanks in part to the exhaustion that was ever present and right below my consciousness. Fern would stand next to me at the side of the table, ask me if there were any acute symptoms that I was experiencing, and then "read" my pulses.

Acupuncture diagnosis is done by placing three fingers on the three pulse points located at each wrist and then sensing different types of pulse beats that occur beneath the practitioner's fingers. Each pulse is associated with a different organ. The practitioner determines the health of each organ, meaning its relative state of balance or imbalance. That information guides the practitioner in how she will treat the client.

Acupuncture is done by inserting very thin needles superficially into the skin. Each needle is placed at precise points along 12 pathways known as meridians. These meridians are channels of energy—an energy known in China as *chi* or *Qi*. The Chinese, like virtually all traditional cultures, believe that the physical body is animated by a life force, or life energy. The Greeks called this energy *pneuma*, or breath; the Hindus called in *prana*; the Chinese call it *chi*, or *Qi*, and Japanese refer to it as *ki*. Each of us has our own unique life energy that in turn is joined to the universal life force, or Great Spirit. Our life force flows along these 12 meridians and thus provides every cell, tissue, and organ with the living power that sustains the physical body with life. This life energy becomes imbalanced due to our lifestyle, thoughts, emotions, and dietary practices. When the life force becomes imbalanced, blockages arise along the meridian. These blockages act like great stones in a river, damming the flow of energy to cells, organs, and tissues. Without adequate life energy, cells become deformed, organs weaken, and sickness arises. Acupuncture points act as generators of life energy. By inserting a needle into the acupuncture point, the practitioner stimulates the point and triggers an increased flow of energy along the meridian and to the organ. This is meant to overcome the imbalance in the pathway and optimize the flow of chi to the organ, thus restoring it to health. Later on, I would learn that there is a considerable body of scientific evidence to support the practice of acupuncture in the treatment of many illnesses and conditions. I knew nothing of this evidence at the time. For me, acupuncture was yet another way that I was trying to help myself get well.

At the very least, I felt blessed to be in Fern's company. Her kindness, sensitivity, and love made me feel seen by someone wise and knowing. And the acupuncture made me feel good. Every time I left Fern's office, I felt a little lighter in body and spirit. Something inside of me told me that acupuncture was good for me, though there were no overt changes in my condition. But that was enough for me. More and more, I was turning to my inner voice for counsel and guidance. I was also turning increasingly to people who supported my life, as opposed to those who were trying to kill the cancer and, in the process, kill me, as well.

In August, I completed radiation treatment and then began the second phase of my chemotherapy protocol. This one, which was to last until October, would require me to take Taxol, another chemotherapy drug that also caused intense side effects, though different from my original chemotherapy regime. Taxol caused intense rheumatoid arthritis symptoms. My wrists, elbows, shoulders, hips, knees, and ankle ached so intensely that I could barely move my body. Once the effects of the Taxol took hold of me, I could do nothing but get into bed and writhe in pain. I often wondered, as I lay in bed in agony, how people with severe rheumatoid arthritis survived the disorder. Such intense pain brought me to the limits of my will to survive and made me see the blessing that was death.

My doctor prescribed Decadron, an anti-inflammatory, which did relieve most of the pain, but left me feeling stiff, achy, and vaguely old and creaky in my bones. The Taxol also caused my red and white blood cell counts to fall dramatically. To raise them, I had to inject myself in my hip with two drugs, Nupogen and Epogen, every day for a week after each chemotherapy treatment. I was told by a nurse that each shot cost somewhere between $700 and $1,000. Many of my chemo buddies joked that there must be traces of gold in the medication!

Meanwhile, I was undergoing regular blood tests and check-ups by Dr. Meredith. I also saw a specialist, and the news was never good. At one meeting, I asked her if she thought that I should have my left breast removed as a way of preventing the cancer from emerging again. No, she said. It wouldn't do any good. In all likelihood, the cancer would come back within a year in the area of the right breast, even with the mastectomy. The oncologist told me flatly that the chemotherapy was not working. If I had any chance of living, I would have to undergo tamoxifen treatment.

But then a serendipitous encounter planted a seed in me that would ultimately change the course of my treatment. In mid-October, at one of Lisa's cooking classes, a friend of mine named Louise Sharp told me that she was following a "healing" macrobiotic diet, meaning a diet that was much more specifically designed for her condition. Louise is a beautiful, loving, and charming Italian woman. But now, more than ever, she visibly glowed with good health.

"Who gave you this healing diet?" I asked Louise.

"I saw Warren Kramer for a consultation," Louise said.

Warren Kramer, who at the time was in his mid-30s, was a macrobiotic counselor with a lot of experience working with gravely ill people. I asked Lisa how I might see him. Lisa responded by telling me that Warren would be coming to her house to provide personal counseling the following week. I wasted no time in arranging a consultation with Warren.

The following week, we met in the afternoon in a windowed alcove in Lisa's living room. Immediately upon meeting Warren and shaking hands I sensed that he was serious, capable, and sincere. Warren took a picture of my face with a Polaroid camera and then carefully examined my face, the sclera of my eyes, and the underside of my forearms. He focused intensely as he examined me. Once he was finished, he sat back in his chair and outlined the diet I should follow.

I had already been following a clean macrobiotic diet, free of any dairy products, red meat, chicken, or eggs. I ate cooked whole grains, especially brown rice, three times a day. I ate lots of green vegetables, especially the crucifers—broccoli, cabbage, collard greens, kale, and watercress—and roots. I also ate beans, sea vegetables, and soups, especially miso soup, which I had every morning.

Warren gave me a booklet that listed all of the foods and numerous recipes. He explained the diet that I should follow in meticulous detail, going over every grain, vegetable, bean, sea vegetable, condiment, and soup. He said that I should eat brown rice, barley and millet—those three should be my staple grains. But he emphasized certain dishes that I should eat regularly. As it turned out, I had been eating none of these foods at that point. Among the dishes that he stressed were dried daikon radish with onions, as well as grated carrot and grated diakon, both mixed together. I later learned that diakon could break up masses and tumors in the body. He gave me recipes for several specialty dishes that included carrots and burdock. Burdock has long been used as a healing food to strengthen the kidneys. He recommended a recipe for shiitake mushrooms and kombu seaweed, which have powerful anti-cancer and immune boosting properties. He also told me to eat black soybean stew, with vegetables, which would also promote the health of my kidneys. He stressed the importance of kuzu drink, which he said was made from kuzu—the powdered root from the kudzu plant—along with a Japanese pickled plum, called umeboshi. Kuzu is a highly effective thickener. When cooked in water with umeboshi and a drop of tamari, kuzu drink is highly alkalizing, and strengthening to the intestines. Warren said the kuzu drink would help counteract the effects of the chemotherapy. Finally, he described a variety of sea vegetable dishes, all of which, he said, would help boost my immune and cancer-fighting systems.

Warren had recipes for all of the foods he recommended. I had heard that Warren was an excellent macrobiotic cook, and this soon became apparent as he described the step-by-step process in making each dish. He watched me closely as he described the foods and recipes he wanted me to follow, ascertaining whether or not I was actually comprehending what he was saying. In fact, I was gobbling up every detail. Finally, he recommended that I walk every day and do the body scrub, which was to rub my entire body with a moist, hot towel to promote the elimination of toxins from my system.

The more he talked, the more confident and enthusiastic I became. I already believed that macrobiotics would help me, and the more I listened to Warren, with his grounded and painstaking attention to detail, the more certain I was that everything he advised would work.

Years later, Warren shared his feelings about our first meeting.

"The first thing that I noticed when I met Meg was how weak and swollen she was from the chemotherapy," Warren recalled. "That was my first concern. I gave her a lot of different dishes to strengthen her and help rid her body of the chemotherapy. But the thing that really struck me about Meg was her spirit. She had the most amazing attitude. She was willing to do whatever she needed to do to get well. At that point, I thought, 'Yeah, she can do it. Meg can get well.'"

Warren and I agreed that I would consult with him every other month. He also came regularly to Lisa's house to provide lectures, cooking classes, and personal counseling. From that point on, Warren became my guide.

A FINAL BREAK ∘ That November, I began taking tamoxifen, a drug that is used to treat breast cancer by blocking the amount of estrogen in a woman's body. Estrogen, the female hormone, is a primary fuel for breast cancer. By blocking the estrogen, doctors hope to deprive the cancer of some of what it needs to survive. But none of this sat right with me. The first round of chemotherapy already plunged me into menopause. My ovaries were no longer producing estrogen. I knew that body fat produced some estrogen, as well, but I had no body fat left. By the time I finished chemotherapy, I had lost even more weight, which made me a walking skeleton. I had no muscle left on my arms and little on my legs. If my estrogen levels were so low, why should I be taking tamoxifen? I wondered.

Tamoxifen, I soon learned, was incredibly toxic. There were an array of severe side effects, including internal bleeding, digestive disorders, the possibility of stroke, heart attack, and the recurrence of cancer.

I took my first dose of Tamoxifen in November under the supervision of a doctor, Jane Wingate. Strange things began to happen to me when I started taking the drug. I became intensely disoriented and dizzy, as if I were leaving my body. I forced myself to focus and stay alert. Suddenly, the muscles in my right leg began to cramp. I worked my leg to try to release the cramp, but it remained locked in pain. The pain gave me something to focus on, which kept me anchored for awhile in my body. But soon the disorientation became worse. The room rolled over with every move of my head and I became intensely afraid, not knowing where the symptoms might lead and what might happen to me. I became nauseated and weak, but soon I fell asleep.

The next day, I got out of bed and took a bath. In the bathtub, I did my daily hot towel body scrub with a warm, wet washcloth. This is a commonly recommended practice in macrobiotics. The idea was to gently, but firmly scrub the body so that toxins and other waste products could be eliminated through the pores. To my horror, soon after I started the scrub, my skin began to slough off and the capillaries below opened and began to bleed. I stopped scrubbing immediately, got out of the tub, and gently toweled myself dry. Shaken, I called Dr. Wingate. Could my platelets be low as a result of the tamoxifen? I asked her. Unlikely, she said. Still, I wondered if I had been given too strong a dose of the drug, especially given my weight. How heavy were the women in the research studies, I asked. Were they 200 pounds, 150, even 125? I weighed less than 110 at that point. She didn't know, she said, but brushed aside the question. It wasn't important. I had been given the right dose, Dr. Wingate insisted.

A few days later, I called Dr. Rock at a university medical center, and asked him about the tamoxifen. He told me that many of the women in the research studies could not tolerate the drug's side effects and dropped out of the trials. And then he dropped a bomb on me. He told me that the trials did not show much of a survival benefit for those who took the drug versus those who did not.

I hung up the telephone and wanted to cry. Deep inside, I knew that the tamoxifen would kill me if I continued to take it. I had reached the end of the road with modern medicine.

That night, after Tom came home, I told him that I was thinking of discontinuing the tamoxifen. I would turn to macrobiotics as my sole means of treatment.

"Meg, if you feel that strong, then stop it and don't look back," Tom said. "Why put yourself through any more of this," he said. "For what? Another year of life, if that? And what kind of life is that going to be? Maybe macrobiotics is the best way to go."

The next day, I went into Dr. Wingate's office and told her that I wanted to discontinue the tamoxifen. She became ice cold and distant. "The chemotherapy was only part of your treatment," she said. "The tamoxifen is the next stage of treatment."

Dr. Wingate was angry and upset. But inside, my emotions were exploding. Who would take care of me when I had a stroke? Would Dr. Wingate take responsibility for me after I had become incapacitated and lay dying in some nursing home? Whose life was this, anyway?

"No, I'm not going to continue taking the drug any more," I told her. And with that, I walked out of her office and never saw her again.

When I got outside, I felt as if I had been released from prison. My life was finally my own.

8. Choosing life.

Quitting the tamoxifen and stopping all medical treatment for cancer was the most liberating thing I had ever done. It changed me—body, mind, and soul. I took possession of my life. No one was going to make life-and-death decisions for me any more. It was as if I stood up, looked around, and saw life from an entirely new vantage point. And when I looked back at all that I had been through, I realized that everything my doctors were telling me was leading me inevitably to death.

The treatment they were giving me was killing me—perhaps faster than my disease was. My doctors said that these poisons were my only chance at survival. But not one of them gave me any hope of surviving. They assiduously avoided offering me even a hint of hope, which was their tacit way of communicating that I would be dead soon. Meanwhile, they looked at me as if I were some kind of experiment that was about to go very wrong.

The reason I followed their orders, of course, was that I had accepted the medical propaganda that doctors are the only source of a cure. If they didn't have a cure, than none existed. My acceptance of their belief, and the fear it created in me, lay at the bottom of all of my choices. But then the realization finally hit me. None of this was working. They knew it and I knew it. As long as I followed their advice, I was going to get sicker, until I became withered and lifeless, just as my mother had.

Giving up the medical treatment felt like giving up death itself.

Within weeks of stopping the tamoxifen, I experienced a remarkable improvement in the quality of my life. The fog that seemed to permeate my brain gradually started to clear. The bizarre moments of detachment and loss of reality that I had suffered as a result of the drug passed, as well. These symptoms had frightened me, especially while driving, but in a matter of weeks I felt more in control of myself. The tamoxifen had also caused terrible cramping in my leg, but soon after stopping the drug, these pains stopped.

I had been following Warren Kramer's advice to do a hot towel scrub on my body as a way to promote circulation and help speed up elimination of the toxins through my skin. Unfortunately, I had to stop that practice when my skin started to bleed. I had suspected that the bleeding was caused by a low platelet count, but Dr. Winslow dismissed my suspicion as ridiculous. After I stopped the tamoxifen, I went to Dr. Ping and asked him to do a blood test to evaluate my platelets. Sure enough, they were alarmingly low. Then I learned that one of the side effects of tamoxifen was low platelets.

As my symptoms cleared, I started to feel like myself again. Tom and I had bought a house on the ocean, and I would have breakfast on the patio in the mornings and look to the sea. I ate my brown rice and vegetables, and drank my miso soup. On steely gray days, when the wind turned the tops of the swells white, I would experience bouts of sadness for all that I had been through. I wasn't experiencing self-pity—I felt no self-criticism, only a feeling of deep compassion for all that I had been through. Beneath the sadness and compassion lay the bedrock of certainty that what I was doing was right. I drank the miso soup and felt its briny goodness and power enter my body. I chewed my rice 35 to 50 times until it was a sweet liquid that I swallowed as medicine. I did the same with my green and leafy vegetables and colorful roots. Come what may, this was my path and I was finally at peace with myself.

Many of our friends, acquaintances, and the doctors we knew were certain that I had reached the end. Tom wanted both Francis's and Cammie's teachers to know what our children were going through at home in case they suffered lapses in school, or if any social problems began to surface. Tom wrote a lengthy letter to Francis's teacher and explained our situation and expressed his concerns for Francis. The teacher never acknowledged the letter. He then telephoned Cammie's teacher for the same reason. When he got done explaining the circumstances, there was dead silence on the other end of the line. Finally, the teacher made some perfunctory comments and got off the line. People didn't know how to deal with me, or more accurately, with death. A doctor we knew and occasionally socialized with begged Tom to get me to undergo bone marrow stem cell transplant. It was my only hope, she told Tom. Later, she confessed to us that when she heard I was practicing macrobiotics, she thought I was "pathetic."

None of this affected me in the slightest. I was utterly and completely committed to macrobiotics, and I had the deep conviction that it would work. I followed Warren's healing diet with a religious conviction. Even though the chemotherapy, radiation, and tamoxifen had caused substantial weight loss, Warren's recommendations caused me to lose another ten pounds.

I called Warren and asked him about the weight loss. He questioned me closely about my energy levels, appetite, bowel habits, and moods. I explained that I actually felt much better than I had in many months. My energy had significantly improved since giving up the tamoxifen, I told him. It seemed to me that I was eating enormous amounts of food. In any case, I had a good appetite, in part because the nausea that I had experienced on the chemotherapy and tamoxifen had passed. I was not experiencing any digestive problems, either. After suffering from alternating bouts of constipation and diarrhea, thanks to the ulcerative colitis, my digestion had become strong, predictable, and healthy.

"Don't worry about the weight loss," Warren said. "The weight will come back. You're just eliminating the toxins in your fat cells that are supporting the illness."

Warren also explained that the diet would keep my estrogen levels down. He told me that body fat produced estrogen, which was one reason why overweight women had lower survival rates than lean women. The weight loss, in my case, was actually supporting my recovery, he told me. All of this reinforced a feeling deep inside of me that my strength was coalescing.

The diet was having a profound impact on my mood and attitudes, to be sure, but so, too, were the people in the macrobiotic community. Lisa Silverman, Amy Rolnick, Warren, and so many of the people with whom I took Lisa's cooking classes were a constant source of support and positive energy. Fern Tsao, my acupuncturist, was like my Chinese mother. Dr. Ping, who continued to give me vitamin C injections, was a doctor of osteopathy who communicated his belief in my chances of recovering. When I compared the feelings I got from these people, versus those I got from cancer doctors, I realized that my macrobiotic and alternative healers were all sources of hope. My macrobiotic friends and teachers connected with me as a human being. They treated me as if my feelings, and my life, mattered. I was not a dead woman still walking to these people. The medical people saw me as either a lost cause, or, in the case of the doctor touting the bone marrow transplant, a guinea pig with a big insurance policy. Even under the best circumstances, my doctors maintained an impersonal distance from me. In fact, the atmosphere was so professional—a polite way of saying "cold"—that a kind of barrier could be felt against all that might be personal. Sickness and death are intensely personal experiences, of course, but doctors wanted no part of that aspect of clinical care, which is why everything about me was reduced to numbers, charts, medical records, and scheduling. I was a body moving through the system. And the doctors who worked that system wanted me to know that the personal and the emotional part of me were strictly off limits.

The emotion that was most denied in the medical world, of course, is the fear of death. Somehow, the people in the Portland macrobiotic community accepted this fear and were able to get past it. The reason they could do that, of course, was that they had hope. The macrobiotic diet had given them hope. It had also given them gratitude.

We met every week at Lisa's house. Four times a year, Warren Kramer would give a lecture. Lisa would make a big meal for 30 or 40 people, depending on any particular night's turnout. This was Lisa's element. She floated around her kitchen, living, and dining rooms with a big smile and her ever-relaxed manner. Lisa is blessed with a manner that is not only free of pretension, but has a certain way of laughing that pokes holes in inflated egos. And yet, her grounded and practical manner is infused with sincerity. Nowhere did that sincerity emerge in more blessed relief than when she led the community in grace each week. She rarely took a seat when she began the prayer. Lisa, Amy, or Pauline would have made a beautiful meal that would include some type of soup—often sweet squash soup with miso—a delicious grain, or sushi rolls with sliced vegetables and wrapped in nori seaweed, and an array of bright green, orange, and yellow vegetables. All of this would be followed by a beautiful and delicious dessert, oftentimes apple pie that was sweetened with apple juice or rice syrup. We all would be seated at tables spread out in Lisa's living and dining rooms. The meal would be spread out in front of us and on our plates. Clad in her apron, or sweater, with her sleeves rolled up and her hair in slight disarray, Lisa would begin by asking everyone to take a few moments to relax and breathe. "Let's exhale and let out the day's tension," she would say. "Maybe you had a fight with your boss or a coworker. Let it go. You're here now. Just rest. Let's thank the farmers for producing the food we will eat tonight. Let's thank the warm rays of the sun and the soil that grew these foods. Let's thank the insects that helped make the soil rich. Let's thank God, or the power of the universe, or life itself, whatever you want to call it, for bringing us this food. Let's thank each other for being here tonight. Thank you all for coming."

And just like that, everyone felt the blessing. Our hearts opened. Some ate in silence, others ate and talked a little with those around them, but all of us felt uplifted and grateful for the food and each other's company.

After all that I had been through, gratitude now overtook my life. Something shifted inside of me. It was as if a door that had been slightly ajar my entire life was suddenly thrust open and out poured all of this appreciation for my life. And somehow all of these feelings of gratitude landed on…vegetables. Odd as this may sound to someone who had not been left hopeless on the edge of death, I knew, in a deep and visceral way, that these whole grains and vegetables were my salvation. All I could feel was immense and heart-opening gratitude for their every sweet shape and size. I walked down the aisles of the Whole Grocer, my local natural foods store, looked at these foods, and realized that every one of them was full of life.

Life, as an energy or force, had given them their shape, texture, and color. And these foods still held this precious gift. Life burst forth from these wholesome leaves, these penetrating roots, these tiny grains, these orbs of color. Each had its own nature, its own unique way of expressing life. Collard greens, striated with veins, fanned flat and wide. Kale ruffled along its edges. Carrots bravely dug into the darkness of the earth. Celery stood firm and tall. Leeks made delicious rings within rings. Onions shined in yellow or purple light. Squash and pumpkin swelled with the earth's sweetness.

Life flowed down from the heavens and up from the earth and mingled in seeds. It fired these tiny dormant jewels with energy that unfolded into beautiful art forms that were vegetables, grains, beans, and fruits. These foods capture life, I realized, and make it available to me, to those I love, and to the world. As I looked over the long refrigerated produce counter, I said to myself, "I'm so lucky. I can have whatever I want. I'm so fortunate to have macrobiotics."

I filled my cart and bags to the brim. When I left the store, my bags were stuffed with varieties of whole grains, vegetables, beans, and fruit that, before macrobiotics, I never knew existed. They overflowed with greenery. "Wow, my family and I are going to eat all of these vegetables in two or three days," I told myself as I drove away from the Whole Grocer. "And the living goodness in them is going to fill us all with life."

I ate these foods three times a day and watched them change me physically, emotionally, and spiritually. In the mornings, I made miso soup, a vegetable broth that usually contains a seaweed, called wakame, and miso, an aged and fermented soybean paste. Miso is aged anywhere from two months to two years, depending on the type of miso. It is a traditional Japanese food that is used as a base for soups, stews, and sauces. The Japanese like to say that miso "strengthens the weak and softens the hard," meaning that it restores the vitality to tired and sick organs, while softening and dissolving stagnation, cysts, and tumors.

Miso contains a phytochemical called genistein that scientists have recently discovered performs the almost miraculous feat of cutting off blood flow to cancerous tumors, thus suffocating them. This incredible process, called anti-angiogenesis, is thought by many cancer experts, including the renowned Dr. Judah Folkman of Harvard Medical School, to be an ideal form of cancer therapy—one that attacks the cancer cells but leaves normal cells unaffected.

Miso is rich in friendly bacteria, such as lactobacilli, which aids digestion and makes nutrients more available to the small intestine. These bacteria also consume carbon dioxide and give off oxygen, further enhancing the life of the digestive tract. And miso is also a source of protein.

Over the centuries, a folklore about miso developed in Japan. Its legendary powers were only enhanced in the last century, when Japanese physician Tatsuichiro Akizuki, MD, used miso to treat the sick and wounded who had survived the dropping of the atomic bomb upon Nagasaki. Akizuki recorded his experience in a book he wrote after the war.

"On August 9, 1945, the atomic bomb was dropped on Nagasaki," he wrote. "It killed many thousands of people. The hospital I was in charge of at the time was located only one mile from the center of the blast. It was destroyed completely. My assistants and I helped many victims who suffered from the effects of the bomb. In my hospital there was a large stock of miso and tamari [the liquid that comes off the miso during the fermentation process and also used a condiment and soup stock]. We also kept plenty of brown rice and wakame [sea vegetable]. So I fed my co-workers brown rice and miso soup. I remember that none of them suffered from the atomic radiation. I believe this is because they had been eating miso soup."

I had been exposed to a great deal of radiation as a form of treatment. And the chemotherapy felt like a fire in my veins. I had not been a victim of the atomic bomb, but it felt to me as if a bomb had gone off in my life, and like the Japanese of Nagasaki, miso soup was part of my answers, too.

Miso is highly alkaline and has long been used to treat stomach and digestive problems. Its natural alkalinity balances stomach and bile acids that accumulate in the duodenum, the first part of the small intestine. Miso alkalizes the entire digestive tract, thus protecting the life of delicate cells and tissues that exist throughout the small and large intestine.

The macrobiotic diet includes many other fermented foods, including shoyu (all natural soy sauce), tamari (the liquid runoff from miso), tempeh (fermented soybean patties), natto (fermented soybean condiment), pickles, and sauerkraut. All of these foods alkalize the blood and strengthen organs, including the spleen, large intestine, and kidneys. In traditional Chinese medicine (TCM), the spleen is regarded as the governor of digestion. It sends life force, or *Qi,* to the entire digestive tract, but particularly to the large intestine, and in this way strengthens the large intestine. Miso also strengthens and tonifies the kidneys, making the organs more fit and vital. As I would later learn, this would be fundamental to my transformation.

I would add a spring onion and another vegetable, often a green, such as kale, or broccoli, to my miso soup and then garnish it with parsley.

In addition to my miso soup, I ate a grain, such as brown rice or oatmeal, and then another two vegetables. I tried to get nine servings of vegetables each day, which was never a problem for me. Serving size didn't matter and I could eat as much as I wanted of all of these foods.

Lunch was usually leftovers from the previous night's dinner. I would eat a whole grain, such as brown rice, barley, or millet—these were my staple grains—and whatever leftover vegetables I still had. Usually I would boil or steam a fresh vegetable, as well.

Dinner included a bean, usually chickpeas or black beans, lentils or aduki beans. Very often I pressure cooked the beans with other vegetables, or boiled them with a sweet vegetable. I loved aduki beans that were boiled with a sweet butternut or acorn squash. Whenever I made beans, I soaked them overnight, threw out the soaking water, and then added new water to the pot. I also added a stalk of kombu seaweed, which added minerals to the beans, and helped make them softer and more digestible.

I pressure cooked brown rice often, but I also boiled it. Brown rice and other grains were the center of my meal. Usually I soaked the rice overnight to make it easier to cook, more delicious, and more digestible. When I cleaned the rice before cooking, I sometimes recalled my years in Korea and how my cleaning lady, Miss Choi, whom we called Ajama, or grandmother, would wash her rice with such care before cooking it. I mimicked her now. I poured rice into a pot and then ran cold water over it, holding the grains in my hands as the water in my sink cascaded down upon it. I imagined that I was putting my own loving and grateful energy into the rice as I held each handful. Then I stirred the rice counterclockwise, pouring off the cloudy water, filling it again, and again, until it was clean.

I boiled or pressure cooked beans, chopped a squash and boiled or baked it, and then chopped a variety of roots, greens, and leafy vegetables and either steamed or boiled them. I made exotic vegetables, such as lotus root, with its tiny holes embedded throughout the gourd-like vegetable, and burdock, a long tough root that has been used by traditional healers for centuries to strengthen the kidneys. I made pressed salads with napa cabbage, carrots cut into matchsticks, and red radishes, all lightly sprinkled with sea salt.

All of this cooking produced smells that were so earthy, so different, and so exotic that they changed the atmosphere of my house entirely. I walked into my house after shopping and was immediately confronted by the new smells of macrobiotic cooking. The smells were clean, powerful, slightly acrid, and definitely comforting. This was a new culture, a new way of living. It was like being invited into another world, one in which the rules were entirely different, and the possibilities endless.

I bought a bunch of cookbooks, including *The Book of Whole Meals*, by Anne Marie Colbin, *Rice is Nice*, by Wendy Esko, and *The Self-Healing Cookbook* by Kristina Turner. I spent hours thumbing through the books, reading about the foods, and learning how to make them. Everything was entirely new to me. At times, I felt as if I were being reborn into a new world.

Cleaning and cooking grains and vegetables, reading cookbooks, and learning about the medicinal effects of each food—this was my daily practice. It was a kind of meditation on healing and health. It gave me a practical and grounded set of activities each day, all of which were geared toward one thing: giving me back my life, and restoring my family.

I became so enamored with the beauty of vegetables that I wanted cups, saucers, plates and bowls that were decorated with vegetable art. Much to my surprise, they were exceedingly difficult to find. There were the occasional porcelain carrots or eggplants on cups, but whole sets of dishes, or simply cups with colorful vegetables on them were rare. I decided to make my own art with vegetable designs. I made silk screens of radishes and carrots, beautiful pea pods, and snow peas. Then I placed these images on aprons for Lisa with the words 'Five Season's Cooking School' emblazoned on them. I also made t-shirts with the same art and lettering and gave them to Lisa to give to her helpers. My burst of creativity, and the art that flowed from me, felt like a sign that my life force was returning. It was too early for me to celebrate anything, but I was aware that my enthusiasm for life was entirely new and completely out of character with the long death march that I had been in. There were others symptoms of restoration. My energy levels gradually got stronger. I could do more during the day and didn't need to rest as frequently. I also slept deeply at night, without sleeping pills. My anxiety, which had plagued me for years, began to recede. As the weeks passed, I felt more deeply rooted in my body, more solidly grounded within myself. I was engaged in an entirely new realm of study. In short, I was feeling better than I had been in years.

When I saw Warren Kramer for my regular evaluation, I could hardly contain my appreciation for the diet and his guidance. Warren made small adjustments in what I was eating, but left little doubt that I was well on my way back to health.

As he would say in 2005, "I was very impressed with how much Meg had recovered between our first two visits. Her improvement in just a few months amazed me. Not only did she look great, but she had this amazing spirit. Meg was going to every class she could. She was getting support, and she was reading everything about macrobiotics and health that she could put her hands on. She I was really confident that she was going to make it."

Tom was as amazed as I was. For years, Tom believed, as I did, that chemotherapy and radiation treatment was the only real course of treatment. There was no alternative. The very word alternative meant sham, empty promises, and charlatanism. But as he saw me dying, and realized that the doctors were not giving me one bit of hope, he came to the conclusion that we had to find another way if I was to have any chance of survival.

Now, for reasons that made no sense to Tom, I was suddenly improving. He was happy with my progress, but he didn't quite know how to deal with me, and all the changes I was going through. In reality, I was racing into macrobiotics. I had changed my diet entirely, but I had also introduced us to a whole new set of people who had very different ideas and points of view. They talked about yin and yang, the healing effects of different foods, their own illnesses or conditions, how they came to macrobiotics, and what affects the diet and lifestyle were having on their lives. Like me, many of these people could talk about little else but their new ways of living. To someone who was suddenly plunged into this world, especially for someone who was healthy and living a largely conventional American life, the change must have felt like being dropped into a kind of Wonderland. For me, the world was finally right side up, but for Tom, the world had suddenly been turned on its head.

As always, he managed the white rapids as best he could and made few demands on me as I pulled the family into this new world. In those latter months of 1999, Tom adopted the macrobiotic diet to the extent that he could. He ate what I ate at dinner and then he ate whatever else he wanted the rest of the day. Even before I made obvious improvements in my health, however, Tom saw my commitment to this path and he respected it from the start. This was the way I wanted to live the rest of my life, and if that was only a few more months, than he would walk it with me.

Francis and Cammie took their cues from Tom. I explained as best I could that we were eating this way for our health and that it would make us all much happier. I kept more familiar foods in the house for them and occasionally made organic meat, if they wanted it. But dinnertime was dominated by macrobiotic foods. They watched their father accept the food and listened to him encourage them to do the same. They knew that this was my diet, and if Tom was part of that now, than they had no choice but to be part of it, too.

Still, I wanted them to enjoy the food—that was the only way they would continue to eat this way, I realized. So I came up with recipes that combined macrobiotic foods with those that Tom and the children recognized as "normal."

One of my favorites was a tofu stir fry that included organic, marinated chicken to ease the transition. The chicken was marinated in tamari, a soybean product that's rich in healthy flora and substances that fight cancer; fresh, grated ginger juice, which promotes intestinal and liver function; mirin, a rice wine sweetener; and oil. Tofu takes on the taste of whatever you marinate it in, so it ended up tasting like the chicken. In addition, I served brown rice topped with vegetables—usually sautéed carrots, onions, broccoli, snow peas, and shiitake mushrooms. To my great satisfaction, they loved the tofu. My children couldn't tell the difference between the tofu and chicken, and regularly asked for more tofu. Francis would bring his plate to the stove and take more tofu from the pan. And when no more tofu was left, he would sneak it from other plates at the table.

This dish became a weekly favorite that I served with miso soup and steamed greens. And in time, they came to enjoy the tofu so well that I no longer had to add chicken.

I had to constantly find ways to get my children to eat green vegetables. Cammie would eat anything healthy—she was young, flexible, and seemed to have a natural wisdom when it came to the food—but Francis resisted, which occasionally forced me to succumb to bribery. Usually, the bribe was dessert—"If you eat all your collards greens, you get the strawberry crisp I made," I would say. And sometimes I told them I would pay them to eat their greens. One day I bribed Francis to eat all his kale and when he was done, I was so happy that I said, "Francis, you made my day."

"Mom, you lead a really boring life," he replied.

We both laughed out loud, but secretly I told myself that I was lucky to have a life.

Gradually, Tom and the children came to enjoy the macrobiotic foods more and more. I knew that as I learned to prepare these foods, we would come to think of macrobiotics as the most enjoyable—not to mention the healthiest—way to eat.

In fact, that's eventually what happened. As my children got older and more secure in themselves, they came to accept their diets as normal, delicious, and even a more intelligent way to eat. When Cammie was in the fourth grade, her health teacher told the class that they should drink two-to-three glasses of milk every day to get enough calcium. Cammie told the teacher that her family did not drink milk. Instead, we ate kale, collards, and other green vegetables, which had just as much calcium as milk did. Moreover, the calcium was in the vegetables was easier for the body to absorb. Shocked, the teacher looked at her and exclaimed, "What, you mean you actually eat that stuff?" She replied, in a matter of fact way, "Yes, and sometimes I eat it for breakfast!"

Needless to say, I was very proud of her when she told me about this incident later. Cammie could be different, without feeling inferior. I realized that my daughter had learned lessons in childhood that I was only learning now.

Though Tom and the children could stray from macrobiotics anytime they wanted, I was strict with myself. I never ventured beyond the standard diet—not a single time. This was my life now, and the more I ate whole grains, beans, and vegetables, the more I craved these foods.

That fall, the Portland macrobiotic community had a holiday potluck feast at my house. About 45 people showed up with great platters of gourmet macrobiotic foods. There were endless spreads of grain-and-vegetable salads. Macrobiotic versions of Waldorf salads, Caesar salads, tabouli, and antipasti. Huge bowls of brown rice, quinoa, barley, all mixed with colorful vegetables, many garnished with various kinds of sauces. There were endless varieties of sushi rolls. Some were made with soba, or buckwheat noodles, with pickled vegetables in the center and wrapped in nori seaweed. There were soups, tofu dishes smothered in mushroom-and-tamari sauces, fried noodles with vegetables, and fried grains and vegetables that were combined with sauerkraut. People found ways of making beans that I never dreamt possible—sweet and sour bean dishes, spicy beans, beans and squash, beans and vegetables, and beans and rice. And then there were the vegetable dishes! Every conceivable vegetable seemed to be on display, all made a little differently—boiled, baked, steamed, and sautéed in olive or sesame oil. The colors made rainbows on my table. And finally, there were the desserts—fruit pies, jello-like kantens made with fruit and apple juice, puddings made from kuzu, and a variety of juice and rice-syrup sweetened desserts, such as blueberry apple crisp, and adzuki bean brownies.

When the food was placed on my long table, my sister, Liz, and I stood back and marveled. We recalled the Thanksgiving feasts my mother made and how she spent days preparing and hours cooking the food. We talked about how she had to have a surplus of potatoes—"20 pounds of potatoes!" I said to Liz. "Mom never had enough potatoes!" We both laughed. There was the turkey, of course, other meats, auntie's special bread stuffing, and many varieties of fudge, pies, and ice cream. "Remember how mom used to work for days and then everyone would eat for 15 minutes and then be too full to go on eating?" I asked. "People would have to move away from the table and stretch or take a nap. The food was too heavy for their bodies. It made them sick!" Liz and I couldn't contain ourselves as we thought of those people having to labor to get away from the table.

"Within 20 minutes, they'd be moaning," Liz said.

"Yeah, they'd be asking for mercy and mom would be pushing more food on them," I recalled. "Have some more pie, just a slice. And the slice would be this big!" We both laughed until tears rolled down our faces.

Liz and I looked back over the tables before us. People could eat macrobiotic food and feel satisfied but still feel good. Everyone would go home with platters of leftovers, having eaten their full, and no one would need a Pepto Bismal or an Alka Seltzer. This was an entirely new world, I thought, yet somehow it felt to me like the one we were intended to live in.

9. The way back.

Giving up the tamoxifen meant leaving Dr. Wingate, another blessing for having let go off the drug. But I was now without a doctor. Even though I was now using macrobiotics as my only form of medical treatment, I still felt I needed a doctor to monitor my health and inform me of any medical choices I might face. My criteria for a good doctor had changed radically, however. I needed a doctor who would treat me with respect. I would not tolerate someone dismissing my concerns, while he or she attempted to impose a medical treatment upon me. After Thanksgiving, I searched for such a person and finally decided to see Dixie Mills, M.D., who practiced at Women to Women, a medical center in Yarmouth, Maine, that specializes in women's health.

Women to Women is located in an old Victorian house that has been fully restored and refitted to suit a very active medical practice. It was founded by a group of women, one of whom remains its co-owner, Marcelle Pick. Marcelle, a nurse practitioner, is in her early fifties. She is strong, confident, and exceedingly competent. She's warm and friendly, someone you instantly respect, yet feel drawn to. People who are treated at Women to Women talk about the respect they are given. Every question is answered, every issue addressed.

The house reflected the women who worked there, especially Marcelle. There were live plants all around the house and fresh flowers in every room, it seemed and lace curtains hung in the tall windows. The ceilings were tall and a great staircase led to the second floor. A beautiful dining room with a long, burnished table served as the place where everyone gathered for lunch and meetings. Bookcases line many of the walls. As I waited to see Dr. Mills, I browsed the shelves, seeing books on every form of alternative medicine imaginable, including macrobiotics. There were many books on spirituality, as well, including Buddhism and other traditions. The entire house was filled with a warm, cozy feeling. There was something intangible about these old houses, I realized. I felt the character of the house embrace me like a loving mother. The women had made a home of their offices. I felt that wherever I might sit down, I could stay for hours.

My initial meeting was with Marcelle, who led me through a series of intake questions about my health and lifestyle. When she was done, I was led to Dr. Mill's office. Dixie Mills, a surgeon who specializes in women's issues, especially breast cancer, is in her early-50s. She is a little quiet, but friendly and supportive. There's not a trace of arrogance in her manner.

We went over my intake chart. I explained the treatment I had had to that point. I then told her that I had decided to go off tamoxifen. I explained the symptoms I was suffering and that I felt the treatment itself was killing me.

To my surprise, Dr. Mills said she agreed with me. Tamoxifen isn't a cure, she told me. Its only purpose is to extend life, but it doesn't do that for everyone. In many people, the side effects far outweigh the benefits. She speculated the drug was probably interfering with the estrogen receptors in my brain, which might cause the kind of loss of reality and out-of-body experiences I was having. I was already in menopause, which meant that my estrogen levels were low to begin with. The tamoxifen would block the receptors in the breast, she said, which would obviously result in side effects.

Dr. Mills told me that she would monitor my blood and my overall condition, but there was no test that could definitively tell me the status of my breast cancer. She then described the AMAS cancer test, which is a blood test that measures AMA, or anti-malignant antibody, a protein created by the immune system that appears when the body is fighting cancer. The test is not 100 percent accurate, she said, since sometimes people with cancer have low AMAS tests. Still, it was worth doing. It would be part of the blood panel she would run on me.

I told Dixie Mills about the macrobiotic diet I was on and my belief that it could help me overcome my cancer. Again, she surprised me by saying that she thought the macrobiotic diet was a good thing and that it certainly might help me. Immediately, she communicated to me that she respected macrobiotics. She said that she knew it had helped other women.

Everything Dixie Mills said was supportive of me personally. She was seeing me, supporting who I was and what I was doing. She wasn't trying to impose something on me, as so many doctors had tried to do before. I needed a doctor who was more my partner in my recovery, not an authority figure who wanted to dismiss my feelings and thoughts. As Dixie would say years later, "Meg struck me as someone who was grounded, practical, and was trying to do everything she could to beat her disease. I felt good about all that she was doing. We don't have a cure for breast cancer. Therefore, there has to be more the patient can do to help herself overcome this disease. A lot of things that people might do for themselves are being denied or suppressed because these approaches don't fit into the standard medical model. Doctors simply don't know about these things, so they dissuade their patients. But you cannot come to work every day and stay positive if you're just working with standard cancer treatment. People have to help themselves and there's a great deal they can do. Meg was doing what she believed to be right and part of my job was to support her, especially when I believed in what she was doing, too."

Perhaps because I immediately felt a rapport with Dr. Mills, I decided to take a risk.

"Tell me that you believe that I can cure myself with macrobiotics," I said to her.

"I believe that women can heal themselves with diet," she said sweetly.

"No," I said. "Tell me that I can cure myself with diet."

"I think you can," Dixie Mills said.

"Thank you," I said. "I really needed to hear that from a doctor."

SIGNS OF RECOVERY ○ Throughout the fall of 1999, small blessings occurred for which I was very grateful. For one, my hair started to grow back. It came in soft and curly, almost like a baby's, except that it was salt and pepper. Also, my blood platelets returned to normal, which meant that I could resume my hot towel scrub.

Each morning, I filled the sink with hot water, dipped a white cotton wash cloth into the water, rung it out, and began scrubbing my entire body. I started scrubbing the fronts of my both hands, and then the backs, and then went to my neck. From there I scrubbed my entire torso, paying particular attention to the areas where lymph nodes are concentrated—the underside of my arms, armpits, and groin. I went down my leg and again focused a lot of attention at the backs of my knee, another area where lymph vessels and nodes are concentrated. Finally, I thoroughly scrubbed my ankle and foot, especially the bottom of the foot. In all, it took about 15 minutes and I did it twice a day for the next two years.

For me, the hot towel scrub was something of a marvel. It made my skin glow. In fact, I could always tell if other macrobiotic people in my community were doing the hot towel scrub, because they had that same glow. But it also made me feel calmer, more centered in my body. It was an exercise that gave me more energy and made me feel physically stronger, and of course it improved my circulation immensely. It also promoted elimination of toxins through the pores. And finally, it made me warm. In the past, I had always been cold, especially in the fall and winter, but we made our way toward the end of 1999, I felt myself growing hardier and more resistant to the elements.

These were not the signs of illness, I was certain. I had been sick for too long to be confused about the signs. My growing confidence allowed me to give myself two presents that Christmas.

The first was that I got rid of the chemotherapy port in my chest. I had kept the port for months after I stopped the chemo because I had been getting vitamin C injections directly into my blood stream through the port. But my macrobiotic training had taught me that high doses of vitamin C were very yin, or expansive, which was probably not a good idea at this stage in my treatment, especially since I was getting plenty of antioxidants from my diet.

Dr. Meredith removed the port at her office. The procedure was remarkably simple and no anesthesia was necessary. She simply removed the plastic tube from my chest and gave me a couple of stitches to close the wound. But what a victory it was for me! Not many people get rid of their ports, I told myself. In fact, I bet that a lot of people die with those ports in their chests, I speculated. This is a milestone. This is a big step on the road to recovery. Good-bye chemotherapy. Good-bye cancer, I told myself. Good-bye to all that.

Dr. Meredith had not encouraged me to get rid of the port, and treated my decision with the same abstract detachment with which she always engaged me. She didn't congratulate me or share my feeling that this was a small but significant victory in my recovery process. I figured that she probably thought that she'd have to put it back in at some point.

The other gift I gave myself was to throw away my commode. I had kept it close to my bed because I could not get up and walk to my bathroom. I also needed it to vomit in after my chemotherapy treatments. Over the months, the commode had become a symbol of suffering and of the dying process. I threw it out. Merry Christmas. Happy New Year.

That spring, the necrotic vessels in my hands became normal and more youthful again. My hands had become nearly black with necrosis. Now the skin was turning pink and the vessels soft and blue again.

Meanwhile, I kept returning to Dixie Mills. I saw her every six months, and every time we met, she was a beacon of support and light. It was no surprise to me that my AMAS tests were coming back negative for cancer. Dixie looked at this as merely another piece in a larger picture that was slowly coming into clarity. The picture was health.

"Meg looked good," Dixie recalled years later. "She was very diligent with her diet, which is made up of really healthy foods. And she was following a very healthy lifestyle. I saw my role as supporting her, but also there was a kind of de-hexing going on between us. Meg had been given so many negative messages about her condition and her prognosis. And those messages can have a very powerful and very negative impact on people. They start to believe in the worst case scenario, because doctors are telling them that that's what's going to happen. And that's a kind of hex that is put on people. The word of doctors is taken into the heart and becomes a self-fulfilling prophecy. So we had to turn that around.

"We underestimate the power of hope, I believe," Dixie continued. "You don't want a patient to go off in the wrong direction, and you cannot give hope to someone you feel is doing that. But Meg was not living in some airy-fairy world. What she was doing was practical; her feet were on the ground, so there was a basis for hope. And I had no trouble encouraging her and supporting her hope."

Dixie said those words some five years later, but I could feel her believing in me and supporting me when the outcome was still a question mark. It made a huge difference to be able to talk to a doctor who respected what I was doing and was encouraging me. I also saw that it was a characteristic of Dixie's to be curious about people, and to respect what they were doing to help themselves heal. She was non-judgmental. It almost seemed at times that we were investigating this process together. Meeting with Dixie became a life-affirming encounter, one that I looked forward to, as opposed to dreading.

PROFILES IN VICTORY ○ By the summer of 2000, I knew in every fiber of my being that I had turned a corner. I was off all medications for the first time in more than a decade. My health, from every physical symptom and medical test, was excellent. Yes, there was still a theoretical chance that the cancer might return, but I had learned from my macrobiotic training that food was part of the reason that cancer came back after it was forced into remission. For more than two years, I had been eating a diet that had transformed my health in every way. I had experienced the long decline toward death that was cancer. Since stopping the medical treatment and adopting the macrobiotic healing diet, I had experienced exactly the opposite. I felt deep within my soul that I was free of cancer.

That August, I attended the annual Kushi Institute Macrobiotic Summer Conference that was held at Westfield State College in Westfield, MA. More than 400 people from all over the country attended that year's conference. It was a giant gala celebration of macrobiotic education and I reveled in it.

At one point in the Conference, Phiya Kushi, son of Michio and Aveline Kushi, the founders of the macrobiotic movement in the U.S., gave a short presentation on his lifetime of eating whole grains and vegetables. Phiya was 40 years old at the time. One Phiya's most striking characteristics is his humility. Another is his charming laugh, which bubbles up and out at the slightest provocation. As the son of Michio and Aveline, Phiya has in many ways, lived outside the American culture. He told us that he had never eaten dairy food or any types of meat. When he said this, he gave a shy little laugh, as if he was amused by the curious twist of fate that life had presented him. Then he said something that deeply affected me. "I have never taken a single drug in my life," he said. Again the humble little laugh. "Not even an aspirin. Of course, I cannot take any credit for that. I have to thank my parents, Michio and Aveline Kushi."

I sat there in awe. For me, drugs had been a way of life. They were an essential part of my survival. Pain killers, antihistamines, various forms of cortisone, anti-anxiety medications, and sleeping pills had become so much a part of my daily experience that I took them for granted. Even to hear about someone who had lived their entire life without drugs was something of a minor miracle for me. It expanded what I perceived was possible in life. My children can go through life without the pain, the fear, and the dependency on pharmaceuticals that I had suffered, I told myself. My eyes filled with tears of gratitude.

From Phiya's talk, I went next to a panel discussion led by women who had overcome various types of cancer through the macrobiotic diet. Three women stood out: Bonnie Kramer, who had overcome breast cancer; Marlene McKenna, who had cured herself of malignant melanoma; and Elaine Nussbaum, who had overcome metastatic ovarian cancer that had spread to her bones and lungs. Both Marlene and Elaine had written books about their recoveries— *When Hope Never Dies*, was Marlene's account, and *Recovery from Cancer*, was Elaine's. Marlene's story was presented to the National Cancer Institute (NCI) and was regarded by the NCI scientists as among the most impressive recovery stories that they had ever heard. Elaine's story was equally remarkable. I had known both women and the details of their healing. Bonnie Kramer's story was new to me. It was also the story that was most like my own.

In 2000, Bonnie was in her late 40s. Vivacious and bubbly, Bonnie was so full of life, energy, and optimism that she was, for me, a kind of living testament to the power of macrobiotics to bring someone back from the brink of death.

Bonnie was diagnosed with breast cancer in 1982. Like me, she had been suffering from fibrocystic breast disease. When her tumor was discovered, she was only 28 years old. In February 1982, she started to suffer severe pain that ran from her left breast down through her left arm. A biopsy showed that the tumor was malignant. A radical mastectomy was performed in which her breast and seven lymph nodes were removed. Six months of chemotherapy followed, as well as six weeks of radiation treatment. She also was given tamoxifen.

During her treatment, her sister, Margaret, gave her an article that appeared in *Life* magazine about Dr. Anthony Sattilaro, then president of Methodist Hospital in Philadelphia, who had been diagnosed with metastatic prostate cancer that had spread throughout his body. After being given 18 months to live, Sattilaro adopted a macrobiotic diet. Fourteen months later, his doctors pronounced him completely free of cancer.

Bonnie rejected the article and continued her medical treatment, which she believed had eliminated her cancer. But in 1983, she began suffering from severe menstrual cramping, stabbing pains, and bloating. Four years later, in January 1987, a bone scan revealed bone cancer in her pelvis, ribs, and spine. She also had numerous tumors in her ovaries and uterus.

Doctors performed a hysterectomy, followed by radiation treatment. She rejected chemotherapy because she couldn't bear the thought of the painful side effects again.

Shortly after she began the radiation treatments, she woke up one morning with the memory of the *Life* magazine article about Dr. Sattilaro. Shortly thereafter she bought a copy of *The Macrobiotic Way*, by Michio Kushi, and adopted the macrobiotic diet.

Bonnie is a very spiritual person, having been raised in a devout Italian family. Everyday, she asked that God lead her to the solution to her illness. She also followed the work of Bernie Siegel, M.D., well-known author of *Love, Medicine, and Miracles*, which reported the mental, emotional, and spiritual links to illness and recovery.

Bonnie did not know how to cook the macrobiotic foods, and hadn't been exposed to expert cooking. She cooked the food on her own and, as she liked to say, made a pretty big mess of it. Unable to eat very much of the food, and still ravaged by the cancer, Bonnie lost a great deal of weight and become extremely weak. Her only hope lay with the diet, but she hadn't yet developed a taste for the food.

From the dais, Bonnie recalled how her friend, Mary Sprague, supported her by adopting the diet herself and would frequently eat with Bonnie.

"Oh Bonnie, isn't this food delicious," Mary would say to Bonnie, hoping to encourage her to eat more. But Bonnie's appreciation for the food was anything but enthusiastic. "I'm gagging on the miso soup and sea vegetables," Bonnie recalled. "I would say, 'Mary, dying is one thing, but starving to death is a hell of a way to go.'"

Three months later, still practicing macrobiotics, Bonnie was awakened in the middle of the night with a terrible pain in her spine. The tumor in her back had become red, hot, and swollen. Apparently, the swelling was pressing on a nerve and causing tremendous pain.

"I didn't know what to do," Bonnie said. "I called Mary and told her what was going on. She reminded me that the macrobiotic philosophy maintained that once you adopt the diet, you start to eliminate, or discharge, the toxins that support the disease. 'Maybe your body is discharging,' Mary said.

"'Oh Mary,' I said. 'What if the tumor is getting bigger and the disease is progressing. I don't know if I can stand this kind of pain.'"

A few days later, however, all the redness, swelling, and pain had disappeared. In fact, there seemed to be no sign of any tumor on her spine.

"That was a turning point," Bonnie said. "After that, I started to feel better and better. My energy levels returned, my skin became brighter and healthier, and I started to gain weight. I felt like I had come through something and I was on the other side."

In September 1987, Bonnie had a bone scan that revealed that her tumors were 25 percent smaller than they were back in January, just nine months earlier. Her doctors could not explain why her condition appeared to be improving. Bonnie recalled her doctor's words: "Bonnie, you look great. You're obviously making progress. How do you feel?"

"Well, doc," Bonnie told him, "If this is dying, I highly recommend it."

A bone scan a year later revealed that her tumors had nearly disappeared and in September 1989, another bone scan revealed no sign of cancer anywhere in her body.

Today, Bonnie teaches natural foods and macrobiotic cooking in the greater Hartford area.

FREE AT LAST ◦ I returned home from the summer conference in a state of utter certainty that I had healed myself of cancer. Dixie and I discussed my condition and by all the signs that she could point to—my blood work and physical signs—I seemed in excellent health.

"There's not a definitive test that we can give you, Meg, that will tell us if you have breast cancer anymore, or if the disease is going to come back," Dixie told me. "There's only one real sign, and that is if you live. The standard is that if you make it to five years, the disease is probably not going to recur, but we don't even know that for sure."

How ironic, I thought to myself. After all of my years of relying on doctors to tell me if I was healthy or ill, and to treat my sicknesses, I had finally reached the point where doctors could do so little for me. They couldn't tell me if I was healthy, and there was no cure if I wasn't. And this is where my long journey with cancer and medicine had brought me—back to myself. Medical doctors knew how to find sickness, but health eluded them. That's why they wanted me to stay on tamoxifen and even chemotherapy for the rest of my life—because once you were sick, you were always sick in the eyes of most doctors. Health is an unknown state of being for doctors. They did not know how to detect it, or what it really looks like, which is why they didn't know when to call off the war. Illness is all that they understand. Health is a mystery.

And that was where I had arrived—in that mysterious state of health where doctors could no longer find me.

The lessons lit up inside of me like a line of street lights that flashed on along a darkened street. I realized that all that my doctors had done for me had actually contributed to my survival. There was no doubt in my mind that the surgery, chemotherapy, and radiation had weakened the cancer and prolonged my life. Without medical treatment, I am certain that I would have died long ago. This realization left me in a state of deep gratitude to all my doctors. But I also knew in my heart—just as they had known in theirs—that all their treatments would not have saved me. Nothing they had to offer was going to stop this cancer. They could weaken it, and give me time, but they couldn't kill it. The conclusion was simple: my body was creating the cancer. As long as those cancer-producing conditions continued to exist within me, I would continue to experience cancer. That meant that had the old Meg survived, the cancer would be alive. In that way, I had been locked in some kind of weird symbiosis with my doctors. I produced the cancer and they kept fighting it back, never able to fully destroy it. If allowed to continue, my cancer and the medical treatment would combine to kill me.

In order to escape this loop of sickness and medical treatment, I had to transform my body. I had to radically alter my internal chemistry, my very blood, so that I stopped producing cancer. And the only way I could have done that is by adopting the macrobiotic diet and lifestyle.

It seemed like some kind of bizarre coincidence that when I had adopted the macrobiotic lifestyle, and took responsibility for my life and recovery, I met a doctor who would support me— not only medically, but in my new-found state of maturity. Dixie Mills welcomed a partnership with her patients. She didn't need to wield power over them. In fact, she admitted to me long afterwards that many doctors prefer a partnership with their patients, if for no other reason than such a partnership has a better chance of succeeding in the face of a terrible illness.

"I'm able to do what I do because of people like Meg," Dixie would say years later. "Meg, and people like her, make my job worth doing."

Somehow, I had been led to macrobiotics by forces that I could only describe as divine. I had been guided by the angels and I had found this lifestyle in my darkest hour. And they had brought me to health and were now asking me to decide whether or not I was healthy. "Don't rely on any outside authority figure to tell you about what you know inside, Meg," they seemed to be saying.

I had come as far as I could with medicine. I would continue to see Dixie Mills periodically for the rest of my life. She was my doctor and I needed a doctor. But I had arrived at a place in my development at which I owned my own judgment. I knew myself and I trusted who I had become.

10. *Turning toward the family — and awakening my own dream.*

People who have had near-death experiences say that they will never see life in the same way again. That's how I felt. I had been this close to death and now I felt physically healthy and more alive than at any other time in my life. My heart opened and out poured all of this gratitude for the second chance I had been given.

My recovery changed the way I saw life, too. I realized how much suffering came from our denatured food and agricultural methods. I saw how overweight women and men struggle with even the simplest tasks, like getting in and out of their cars, or grocery shopping, or walking in the summer heat. Friends confided that they were suffering from chronic heartburn, or constipation, or acid reflux. Newspapers reported the dramatic rise in inflammatory bowel disorders, such as Crohn's or colitis. High blood pressure, arthritis, asthma, and attention deficit disorders were now so common that people hardly mentioned them. It seemed that everyone has a family member with cancer. And more and more people are worried about getting Alzheimer's and Parkinson's disease in their senior years. People think nothing of taking two sets of medications—one for their incurable disorders, and another to reduce the side effects from their primary medications. Unfortunately, the medications don't cure anything—they just reduce the symptoms, if only temporarily. But the drugs have side effects, which mean that most people are trading in one set of symptoms for another. There can be no doubt that much of this suffering, and our drug dependency, comes from the food we are eating.

All of this affected me in the most personal way, however. It aroused my maternal instincts and made me concerned for my children. The thought that Francis and Cammie might have to endure some version of what I had suffered the previous 10 years was too much for me to bear. My fear was heightened by the knowledge that the foods children are eating today are far more toxic than those I grew up on in the 1950s and 60s. Also, I was outraged at our schools, which are among the primary suppliers of these poisons—not only in the cafeterias, but also in the hallway vending machines. The so-called foods that come out of these machines are nothing more than sugar, fat, and synthetic chemicals rolled up in fancy packaging. They are so addictive that they virtually guarantee the food manufacturer a captive market. Food companies are maximizing profits by creating addictions in our children for substances that will destroy their health and lead to unimaginable suffering.

I knew I had to do something, but with all the temptations that children face today, I wasn't sure what I could do.

In the fall of 2001, Francis was 15 and Cammie 11. Tom and I decided to send them private schools in Western Maine. Most students board at the schools they would be attending and eat at the school cafeteria. I could not let that happen, especially during their growing years when they were especially vulnerable. I decided to move to Bethel, a small town close to both of the schools my children would be attending. My plan was to have them live with me and commute to school so that I could cook for them every day. Tom would stay in Cape Elizabeth to be near his work and would make the two-hour drive to Bethel on Wednesday nights and weekends. Things would be a bit inconvenient for a few years, but the plan was doable and worth the sacrifices—or so I thought.

That August, Francis, Cammie, and I moved into a house in Bethel and settled into our new life, and in September the children began school. Each day, I made them breakfasts and dinners at home, and lunches-to-go if they chose. It didn't take any time before we had fallen into a routine that my children took for granted. And they enjoyed the food I prepared. Yes, they occasionally ate foods that were not prepared at home, but those excursions were not the norm. Each day, they ate three good meals, along with healthy snacks and desserts. They were building their bodies from the raw materials derived from whole grains, fresh vegetables, beans, sea vegetables, miso soup, and fruit. And in no time, I could see the results of the food in their beautiful skin, their bright eyes and smiles, and their tremendous vitality. Seeing them healthy and doing well gave me such a deep satisfaction that only a mother can truly understand.

It was not until later that I learned of Tom's resentment of my decision to move to Bethel with the kids. I made the decision and thought it a necessary one and expected his cooperation. I had always supported Tom in his job over the past 20 years by moving when his job required it. Now I expected the same support in my decision. I felt that my job as a parent required me to do this but he supported me reluctantly. As time went on, he resented my decision to do this and was secretly angry about it. He denied this. I later read how sometimes when a person does not admit they are angry about something then they become angry all the time—and it comes out in other ways.

GOING BEYOND MY LIMITS ○ Once our routine was established and running smoothly, I felt the need to do more. If macrobiotics could help me and my family, it could help millions of others, too. Of course, I felt a special desire to help women with breast cancer, but the sheer enormity of the problem made me question whether I could make a difference. What could I do, except to take care of my own family, I asked myself? Besides, I didn't know enough about macrobiotics yet, and Lisa Silverman was already doing a great job. Lisa was so relaxed, comfortable, and competent in front of a group. And people loved her. What qualified me to teach macrobiotics? Then I thought, why *not* me? In fact, I had something that most teachers don't have. I had overcome cancer. I had the experience of cooking and creating a health-promoting lifestyle to save my life. I didn't have to know everything about food and health. And I didn't need to pretend to know. All I had to do was tell people what I did to make myself well, and then let them decide what they wanted to do.

"Be the change you want to see," Mahatma Gandhi said. Those words kept ringing in my ears. I wanted to help people avoid the fate that I had suffered, and to give hope to those who were already ill.

All of these questions were fluttering around inside my mind when Lisa came to me at the very beginning of January 2002 and asked me to teach in her stead at the Cancer Community Center in South Portland. The lecture, entitled "What is Macrobiotics," was scheduled for the end of January. I could hardly believe my ears. At first, all my doubts rose inside of me. "I've never given a lecture, Lisa. I don't even know how," I said. Lisa wouldn't hear my protests. "Do it, Meg," she said. "You have the strength. You have the courage. And you have the experience. Look at what you've done."

I thought about it for about ten seconds and then said, "You're right." As soon as I said it, I was thrilled and nervous at the same time.

I studied for weeks. I read and reread all of my macrobiotic books, including the *The Macrobiotic Approach to Cancer* and *The Macrobiotic Way*, both by Michio Kushi. I reread my cook books and went to websites that offered information about breast cancer and diet. I wrote out my talk and memorized it word for word. On the day I gave my lecture, I brought bags full of vegetables, whole grains, and fruit and placed them on the table in front of me. Twenty people showed up, many of them suffering from cancer. The rest had loved ones who had the illness. I told my story and how I had restored my health. Then I gave a short presentation on how a macrobiotic diet might help people with disease, especially with cancer. As I spoke, I found myself becoming increasingly comfortable telling people what I had experienced, and what they could do to help themselves. When it was over, people gave me a big round of applause. Many came up to me and asked how they could learn more about macrobiotics. I gave out lots of information about the Kushi Institute, where Michio Kushi and other senior macrobiotic teachers taught. But in the back of my mind, I was thinking about ways that I could reach more people myself.

That same month, a massage therapist, June Hemlock, who worked with Dr. Meredith asked me to give a lecture to her support group for people suffering lymphodema, or swelling of the lymph nodes. Many of these people had cancer. I did the same intense preparation for this lecture and it was just as successful as my first one.

A month later, I was invited to do a series of six cooking classes on macrobiotics at the Fair Share Market in Norway, Maine, not far from Bethel. The series was to start in February and run through March. I had to bring all the food and equipment I needed in order to cook. For a woman with only one leg, transporting those things wasn't easy. I made about a dozen trips between my kitchen and the back of my station wagon in the ice and snow, and then another half-dozen from my station wagon to the Fair Share Market. By the time I was ready to give the class, I was exhausted and ready to go to the chiropractor. But I loved it. Again, about twenty people showed up for the class. This time, most were healthy, which thrilled me. This was part of my dream—that strong and healthy people would adopt this way of life and spread it among their friends and peers. If healthy people realized that this food was just as delicious and satisfying as their old diets, they would adopt macrobiotics for the pure pleasure of the food. With little effort, most of the sicknesses we suffer from today would disappear.

My classes took place on Monday or Tuesday nights, depending on the week. The series began with an introductory talk, "What is Macrobiotics?" I then dedicated one whole class to each of the five major parts of a meal: soups, grains, beans, vegetables, sea vegetables, and desserts. The classes were fun and informative. I was watching people change their lives, which gave me such feelings of satisfaction and fulfillment.

When I finished the series, I was asked to do another series of six classes at the Center for Hope and Healing in South Paris, Maine. That series ran from March to April, 2002. And when it was completed, I was asked to come back to the Cancer Community Center in Portland and do a regular, ongoing series of cooking classes, which I have been doing for the past five years. In addition, I regularly assisted Lisa and gave private cooking classes and macrobiotic guidance to people who were sick. More and more people were changing their eating habits and ways of living as a consequence of what I was doing. Many were people with cancer, and several of them made the same kind of progress I had. I felt as if I was part of a process that was saving their lives.

Meanwhile, I began attending the Kushi Institute for training in macrobiotic cooking, nutrition, and healing. And through the Kushi Institute, I came to know macrobiotic people from places throughout the U.S. and around the world.

I got involved in the local American Cancer Society (ACS) and established booths where macrobiotic literature was handed out at ACS conventions. I put up flyers for macrobiotic cooking classes and education at the local natural foods stores, bringing more and more people to the macrobiotic way of life. I felt better than I had in years, and naturally I began to blossom. In a matter of months, my dream of contributing to a better world by teaching the macrobiotic way of life had become a reality. I was doing what I loved, which gave me an enthusiasm for living that I had never known before. A new world had opened up for me, one that was filled with meaning and purpose.

Warren Kramer, whom I continued to see for macrobiotic counseling, gave me one of the highest compliments I had received throughout my entire recovery. "In macrobiotics, we say, 'One grain, ten thousand grains,'" Warren began. "It means that one grain can turn into ten thousand grains, which can feed many people. In the same way, one person can change the lives of ten thousand people. Meg embodied that spirit. She was bringing so many people to macrobiotics, and helping so many people, that I had to encourage her to rest and slow down, because she was giving so much. Her positive spirit infused the entire Portland macrobiotic community with love and supportive energy."

I had found my place in the world, I realized. But there was still an unhealed pain in my life—my relationship with Tom.

THE HIDDEN CONFLICT SURFACES ○ I had been sick for the previous 12 years. That much suffering can destroy even the best of marriages. Neither Tom nor I realized how far apart we had drifted from each other, or how much pain we were both carrying from all the trauma of the past decade. But after my recovery, that pain, like an old sunken barge, started to make its way toward the surface.

We were still committed to our marriage, but neither of us knew how to restore the good feelings between us. Instead, we often experienced a subtle, angry tension when we were together. We didn't know how to address and heal that tension, so we settled into a pattern of avoidance in which we spoke almost entirely about our children and the everyday details of our lives.

On Wednesday nights and weekends, Tom would make the two-hour drive from Cape Elizabeth to Bethel. On those days, both of us would be secretly hoping that things would go well between us. I was looking forward to seeing Tom. I missed him during the week and wanted to be with him. As I went through my day, I would be thinking of ways that we might spend the evening together talking or perhaps go out to a movie. A certain anticipation would be growing inside of me. Unbeknownst to me, Tom would be experiencing similar feelings.

"I had this two-, two-and-a-half hour drive from my office to Bethel," Tom recalled years later. "During that entire two hours, I'm thinking of ways to make my encounter with Meg turn out well.

I'm hoping that I'm going to arrive and one of us is going to say something that will turn things around and make us both feel good."

Neither of us knew what to do with the negative feelings we both felt, and the fears that things would not go well. Hope and anger, love and fear lived side by side within us. Both of us hoped that the other would save the day by doing something loving or supportive that would dispel the tension and fear. But that tension formed a very real barrier between us, a wall that prevented us from reaching out to the other because it was too great a risk.

When Tom arrived home, we greeted each other in hesitant tones. If I was at the sink when Tom entered the house, I would turn toward him and say, "Hi." Tom did the same. He would then go directly to the kitchen counter and sift through the mail. As he rifled through the envelopes, opening some, throwing out others, I could sense the tension in him. He was closed and walled off within himself, unavailable to me. I sensed his anger, which made me angry, too.

Of course, in such an atmosphere, it doesn't take much to deepen the conflict. Sometimes Tom would come into the house and set his briefcase and overnight bag down in the middle of a well-trafficked path in the kitchen or living room. I wanted to keep the space clear and would ask him to put his bags in the closet, just a few feet from where he had placed his bags. "Tom, don't put your bag there," I'd say, or "Tom, can you get your briefcase out of the way?" In an atmosphere in which feelings are sensitive and delicate, that's about all it takes to drive people deeper inside themselves, which is what it did for both Tom and me.

Once we started eating, Tom and I communicated through the children. One of us would ask Francis and Cammie about their school work, their teachers, their latest assignments, their skiing, or about other sports-related activities. Both of our children were passionate skiers and both were on ski teams at their respective schools. Francis had become interested in free style skiing, which involved making acrobatic jumps and aerial flips. Now sixteen and mature beyond his years, Francis also had become interested in film. He'd purchased editing equipment for his computer and was formulating a plan to make a movie about free style skiers. Cammie was one of the better Alpine racers in Maine and had a full schedule of practices and races. Both were doing well in competitions and Tom and I loved to know all the details of their latest skiing adventures. Our children's talents and ambitions were starting to emerge and it was a joy to sit around the table and listen to them talk about what they were doing, and what they wanted to do.

The dinner conversation lightened the mood and, for an hour or so, took Tom and me away from our troubles. Once the meal was concluded and the table and dishes cleaned, Tom and I usually helped the children with their homework. Before we knew it, we were tired and the day was over. Tom and I would have spent little or no time together.

The weekends proved even more problematical, especially for me because I had greater expectations for being together. After all, there was more time on the weekend and therefore more opportunity for us to be alone together. But things didn't work out that way. Tom would arrive on Friday night and then spend the rest of the weekend with the kids, either skiing or going to one or another of their competitions. Because of my mastectomy, I had lost muscle in my chest, which prevented me from skiing. Also, the chemotherapy had thrown me into menopause and then triggered the onset of osteoporosis, which meant that I couldn't risk a fall. Skiing for me was out of the question. Tom would be skiing with the kids, and I'd be home waiting for them to return. But more than anything, I'd be wishing I could be with Tom. He, on the other hand, didn't show the slightest need for me. When he arrived back at the house in the evening, he would retreat into his shell and be unavailable to me. I didn't want him to stop skiing, I told him, I only wanted a day each weekend, or part of a day, that we could spend together.

After weeks of this kind of avoidance, I finally said, "Tom, you're running away from me! You spend the entire weekend with the kids. What about me? Don't I get any time? My friends are with their husbands on weekends, but I'm here all alone. I need a little time and intimacy with my husband."

That, of course, would trigger an argument—but never one that got to the heart of our conflicts, or resulted in a true understanding of our respective feelings and needs.

Another trigger for our disagreements occurred when we went to bed at night. Tom would start talking about his financial concerns or some problem at work. He'd dump all of his troubles on me and then roll over and go to sleep. By then, I'd be tense with worry and unable to sleep. I'd lie awake for hours until I finally fell asleep, or wake him up and yell at him for waiting until we were in bed to confide his concerns to me. I told Tom that it was fine to share his concerns with me, but don't wait until I'm ready to fall asleep. Tell me earlier in the evening when we were both awake and had the energy to deal with the problems.

Tom and I realized years later that this was how we experienced closeness and intimacy. We argued until we were spent and exhausted. Only then would the negativity be cleared enough for us to feel the love we had for each other. At that point, we felt closer and could relax or make love. Arguing was the only path to feeling close to each other, it seemed. It was as if the pain of our inner worlds grew more intense over time and, like a pressure cooker on a high flame, had to be released in order for each of us to experience some degree of balance.

It was no coincidence that we were arguing at night, when both of us secretly wanted to be close and intimate, but neither of us knew how to create it. We didn't know how to reach out to the other and, at the same time, feel safe against our fear of being rejected. So both of us played it safe and remained within our respective worlds, which only made our pain worse—that is, until we fought, cleared the air temporarily, and were able to be close.

Our way of creating intimacy was a kind of Catch-22. Arguing often brought us closer, but it also hurt and weakened any trust we had for each other. Every argument felt as if we had created a fresh wound in each other. And both of us were losing any faith that we could talk or be together without engaging in a fight, causing each other immense pain in the process. Meanwhile, we could never get to the source of our anger. Tom continued to be swallowed up in his introverted anger, and I continued to complain about him for not communicating with me.

My principle complaint was that he wouldn't talk to me, which prevented us from having real intimacy. When I said this to him, he would look at me as if he were utterly baffled. As he would confess years later, "I wasn't sure what intimacy really was. And even if I was able to define it, I couldn't tell you how to create it." The truth was, I didn't know what to do. All I knew was that I wanted intimacy, but I didn't know how to break the ice between us, either.

To my amazement, Tom saw us as a loving and happy couple.

"Do you think we have a good marriage?" I asked Tom.

"Of course we do," he said. And that's as far as it went.

In the summer of 2003, Tom agreed to go with me to the Kushi Institute's Macrobiotic Summer Conference, which was held at one of the resorts in Killington, Vermont. We rented a condominium at the resort and had plenty of time to be together. One afternoon, I decided it was time to have our talk.

Tom and I went out for a walk along a path on the ridgeline in the mountains of Killington. Our condominium was on the ridge. As we walked, we could look far down the mountain and see buildings along the slope and in valley below us. I explained my feelings and essentially gave Tom an ultimatum.

"Tom, we need to start spending more time together," I began. "We need to make our relationship a priority. If that's not what you want, then we need to talk about why you don't want to spend time together. What's the point of staying married?" I asked. Tom's eyes suddenly opened wide and I could see the pain in them. He looked at me as if he were shocked.

A few years later, Tom shared his thoughts about that conversation. "My first thought was, 'If you think you're going to find someone better than me, then go ahead.' But then it hit me. Meg wasn't talking about finding someone else better—she was asking me to be better."

"What do you want me to do?" he asked.

"I want you to be engaged in your own healing, just as I am doing," I told him. "I want us both to work on ourselves and to heal ourselves. I want us to learn how to talk to each other, and understand each other."

"Okay," Tom said. "I'll try."

11. *Facing the pain within.*

Love seeks intimacy. I wanted Tom and me to be emotionally closer and to share our inner lives with each other. That was the kind of relationship I wanted with him. At first, I didn't know how we could create such a relationship, but I was open to being guided to my goal.

In the summer of 2004, I moved back to Cape Elizabeth and Tom and I sold our house in Bethel. Meanwhile, I had been seeing a body-centered healer in Portland by the name of Eileen Beasley. Eileen is in her early 40s, has long brown hair, a lean, healthy frame, and a bright and beautiful face. She is full of energy and wisdom, someone who not only heals the body, but is adept at healing emotional and spiritual issues, as well.

Eileen practices craniosacral therapy, a gentle form of therapeutic touch that enhances the movement of cerebrospinal fluid and electromagnetic energy through the central nervous system and throughout the body. Physical and emotional imbalances cause tension and restrictions within the central nervous system, which in turn affect our physical and emotional health. Craniosacral therapy can reduce and in some cases eliminate these restrictions, allowing spinal fluid and electrical signals to flow unfettered through the spinal column and then throughout the body, thus enhancing organ function and overall health. In addition, Eileen practices other forms of therapeutic massage, which also help to heal physical imbalances and longstanding psychological problems.

Working with Eileen involves lying on her massage table and allowing her to place her hands on your body, usually starting at the head. With very gentle touch, she can open the fluid and energy channels that flow along the spine.

She then places her hands on other areas of the body where chronic tension, symptoms of illness, and old wounds may lie. Eileen channels healing energy into the body, especially into the areas and organs that are in distress—the lower back, for example, or the shoulders, or the solar plexus, or liver.

Places within the body that suffer from chronic tension or illness are often sites where deep psychological pain resides, as well. Whenever a person is suddenly made afraid, or angry, or shocked, he or she experiences a body-wide contraction. As muscles and tissues contract, they hold the biochemistry of that emotion—stress hormones, for example—as well as the emotion itself within the tissues. If the person is made to feel fear repeatedly – as most of us were—the resulting contraction becomes habitual so that the body reacts in the same way each time it is exposed to stressful emotions. That means that tension, emotional pain, and fear get locked into the tissues—usually in the same places within the body – every time the person experiences emotional stress. Often, that accumulating tension can lead to physical disorders, such as chronic digestive problems, headaches, ulcers, low back pain, and many forms of illness.

Eileen, who is blessed with an extremely powerful healing touch, places her hands on these traumatized areas of the body. In a soothing and gentle way, she helps the muscles and organs relax, which allows blood and lymph to flow more efficiently again, especially to the affected tissues. As the tissues relax, trapped energy is released and restored to the overall system. Old emotions and memories associated with traumatic events are also released. As these painful emotions and memories arise, Eileen encourages the person to express his or her feelings. She helps the person re-experience her past. At the same time, she provides love and acceptance for whatever arises. In this atmosphere of love, the person comes to love and accept the feelings and memories that she previously rejected. This is one of the ways we become whole again. Wholeness is the basis for health and self-love.

I went to Eileen initially to help relieve the pain from my headaches, and to grieve the loss of my leg and breast. I had done much work on this issue in the past, but still had some unreleased trauma. With her guidance, and gentle healing touch, I allowed so much pain to emerge, and so many tears to flow again. One day, after a particularly emotional session, I asked Eileen, what she thought was happening to me.

"You're releasing anguish," Eileen said.

Somehow she had chosen the perfect word to describe exactly what I was experiencing. It was more than just emotional pain, and more than the memory of physical loss. It was both the heart and the body crying out from my very cells.

In time, I grew more comfortable with my emotions. The grieving brought me to dark places inside of myself; places that were filled with sadness, anger, and loss. At the same time, Eileen's healing touch channeled loving energies into the places in my body where I was most wounded. She was helping me love and feel compassion for my residual limb, my wounded torso, and my broken heart. She also taught me to trust my body to tell me what it needed, and what I might be experiencing emotionally. She was helping me become whole.

One day I said to Tom, "I think it would be really great for you to see Eileen. She's really helping me. Maybe she can do the same for you."

"I'll give it a try," he said.

It didn't take Eileen long to penetrate Tom's wall of defenses and to find the layers of emotion that lay below. Not surprisingly, the first emotions to surface in Tom were anger and disappointment.

"I was holding a lot of anger—anger over our losses," Tom recalled. "I was angry that Meg had lost a leg and a breast and all that meant to our lives, but I was much angrier over the loss of time. Ten years of our lives were spent dealing with cancer. We had no answers and we were living in terror that Meg might die. We lost our youth to cancer. We couldn't do things that other couples could do. It seemed like some people just glide through life unscathed. Maybe that doesn't happen, but it seemed to me that we had a lot more than our share of pain and trouble.

"Not only did cancer take away so much from us, but it also led Meg to macrobiotics, which at first I resisted. I didn't want to have to change our way of eating and thinking, even though both were causing us misery. I was angry that Meg wanted to change the nature of our relationship, too. I resist change. I'm a much more conventional person than Meg. So I had a lot of anger around having to change, especially after all that we had been through."

Tom and I were being coached to see not only the emotions themselves, but our judgments about having such emotions. Our judgments, we soon realized, were a bigger problem than the actual feelings we had.

"When I realized I had all of these feelings, the first thing I thought was, I shouldn't feel this way," Tom recalled. "Some part of me said it was wrong to be angry at Meg for becoming ill, because she couldn't help being ill. But that's how I felt—cheated, disappointed, hurt, and angry—and it wasn't Meg's fault."

Talking about negative feelings without blaming each other had the paradoxical effect of creating compassion for ourselves and each other for all that we had been through. We learned that we can say that we were angry about what happened to us, without being angry at each other. That was a big step because it allowed us to talk about painful emotions, without our discussions turning into arguments. In fact, just the opposite happened, we felt closer to each other after such talks.

Once he started to work on his emotions, Tom had to face an even deeper and darker question inside himself. Did he love me any more?

"I was afraid that I didn't love Meg in the same way anymore," Tom recalled. "She went from being an object of physical desire to an object of pity. That was a really hard thing for me to recognize and accept, but it was true. During those years when she couldn't get around, when she was tired and weak, I had to constantly remind myself that she was handicapped and not to expect too much from her. But the more I did that, the more my picture of Meg changed. She wasn't the same woman to me. How could she be? In many ways, Meg was still Meg, but she was a much weaker version of the woman I fell in love with.

"So I had to look at that and to see if I really did love her anymore," Tom said. "I had to be willing to honestly explore that question. And the answer I discovered was that I loved her more. Amazingly, Meg had resurrected herself. She found a way to heal herself when every one of our doctors were either telling her to forget it, she was going to die, or that they didn't know, but they weren't willing to give us any hope, either. And then to have the courage to go off the tamoxifen, when her doctors were telling her that it was going to keep her alive, just shows you what kind of strength she has. Meg stood up to all of them and found macrobiotics and took off with it. She was right and the doctors were wrong. She got stronger, more positive, and happier every day. She came back to be this positive and powerful person whom I admired, maybe more than I ever admired her before."

Macrobiotics also gave us a huge advantage when it came to working on our emotional lives. This lifestyle gave us hope that any problem could be solved. I came to believe that if I could overcome cancer, I could restore my marriage and have much more love in my life.

One of the beauties of macrobiotics is that it is grounded in simple, healing behaviors that you do every day. After the macrobiotic summer conference, Tom began eating a healthier diet. He also became a wonderful cook. The two of us often cooked together, and often ate our meals as a family.

The food changed us emotionally, as well, which is exactly what the macrobiotic healers predicted.

As anyone who has adopted a healthier diet knows, eating properly cooked plant foods dramatically reduces physical and emotional tension. Whole grains, vegetables, beans, fruit, and fish are easily assimilated by the body. These foods require so little effort to digest and absorb that they are nearly invisible to the body. Once eaten, they leave you feeling nourished, relaxed, and light. You experience feeling emotionally balanced and mentally clear—an important step toward creating a healthy relationship.

Macrobiotic philosophy, which is based to a great extent on Chinese medicine, goes even further. It maintains that the mind and body are intimately united, and that unbalanced emotions are stored, and often arises from specific organs that have been weakened. For example, Chinese medicine maintains that chronic fear arises from weakened kidneys. Heal the kidneys and you will experience greater courage, confidence, and personal power, both macrobiotic and Chinese healers say. On the other hand, excess anger can arise from an imbalanced liver. Heal the liver and anger and frustration diminish, while emotional stability and balanced self-expression return.

Many of the foods in the macrobiotic diet have been used traditionally to restore the health of both of these organs. To make the kidneys stronger, macrobiotic teachers urge people to eat beans, sea vegetables, brown rice, barley, millet, and small amounts of sea salt. At the same time, we should reduce animal proteins, dairy foods, sugar, and cold soft drinks. To make the liver stronger, macrobiotics encourages people to eat lots of vegetables, especially the cruciferous vegetables, such as broccoli, kale, and collard greens, along with barley, whole wheat, and foods that have a slightly sour taste, such as sauerkraut and lemon. We should avoid excess alcohol, foods that are fatty, and those that have been fried, processed, or contain synthetic ingredients. As the kidneys and liver become stronger, we automatically experience less fear, more security, greater confidence, and far less anger and frustration.

I experienced these phenomena firsthand. In the decade of the 1990s, I lived in constant fear that I would be suddenly stricken with some new illness for which my doctors had no answer. I had been diagnosed with bone cancer at the age of 33, and breast cancer at 41. And in between were innumerable diagnoses that were less severe, but often terrifying. It was as if I lived under a dark cloud that was constantly sending out lightning bolts that struck me when I least expected it.

As I ate the macrobiotic foods, my health stabilized and grew stronger. I experienced a miraculous increase in energy and self-confidence. My mind and my intuition became clearer and I felt a growing sense of personal power and control. I was no longer a victim of seemingly random illnesses. For the first time in my life, I felt a sense of purpose. Macrobiotics had changed my path completely, and my heart was filled with gratitude for this way of life.

As Tom ate the food and worked with Eileen, he experienced a similar transformation. He was clearly more balanced, more patient, and open, especially to me. The angry edge that had become so much a part of him was dissolving. He was always secure within himself, but the food seemed to make him more open to new ideas and new ways of looking at life. Macrobiotics had a kind of revolutionary effect on both of us.

The combination of the food, the macrobiotic philosophy, and the work we did on our emotional lives changed both of us. We softened toward each other. More and more, we were learning to listen to, and honor, our own inner feelings, and to share them with each other. We still experienced conflicts, but we were also learning how to deal honestly and openly with them.

We were also healing. We were letting go of old pain and anger. We were freeing ourselves from the past.

12. *A leap of faith.*

Not all of my pain was receding. My residual limb had been a source of periodic shooting pain ever since I lost my leg in 1990. But 10 years later, the pain became more chronic and intense, which is common for many amputees. Part of the reason was that the muscle and remaining fat on my amputated leg had atrophied, leaving little padding for the nerves at the end of the leg, and the tip of the femur, the large bone in the thigh. The withering of my leg also prevented my prosthesis from fitting properly, allowing it to move more freely against the end of my leg. Without sufficient padding, the nerves and bone impacted directly on the plastic socket of my prosthesis, causing intense electrical pains that often lasted for days on end. The pain continued to escalate until, at the beginning of 2005, I was no longer able to wear my prosthetic leg at all. In fact, I could hardly touch my leg now without setting off terrible shooting pains. The leg had become so sensitive that even gently dabbing it with a towel could trigger violent electrical shocks that would radiate through my entire leg and lower body. It was as if an electric cattle prod was held against my leg. Once triggered, the pain usually lasted two or three days, and sometimes a week. The only way I could get relief was by taking a hot bath and over-the-counter drugs.

I realized early on that this was not just a problem of padding, however. I suspected that I had developed a large neuroma at the tip of my residual limb. A neuroma is a benign tumor composed of nerve tissue. Merely touching it can trigger intense pain and/or numbness. I had been telling my orthopedic specialist, Dr. Richard Roma, of my suspicions for the previous five years, but his reaction to my concerns was to look at me as if I had three eyes. He dismissed the notion of a neuroma and noted in my medical record, "Patient thinks she has a 'neuroma.' Looking back, I realized that he hadn't had much experience with amputees. I had grown used to this kind of treatment from doctors, and knew there would be no answers from him.

I also knew that I couldn't live with this pain. I had to do something, but I didn't know what to do. I told myself that I have been here before—lost for solutions and needing to open to divine guidance. *I need help, God,* I prayed. *I'm open. Please give me an answer,* I pleaded. I asked for grace.

I was in limbo, without any sense of what I might do. No inspiration and no intuition came. I was stuck. One day in early-February 2005, I just happened to come across a video in my bookcase that my prosthetist, Bob Hougland, gave to me two years earlier. The tape described the Ertl reconstruction technique, a surgical procedure designed to restore strength and relieve pain in amputated limbs. It is performed by Dr. Janika Ertl, an orthopedic surgeon at Kaiser Permanente in Sacramento, California.

I hadn't looked at the tape. In fact, I resisted even thinking about it. As every amputee knows, the thought of having another operation on a severed limb is horrifying. My greatest fear, of course, was that another surgery would only make matters worse and cause me even greater pain. And my history with doctors made me even more resistant. On the other hand, I knew I couldn't go on living with this pain.

The video tape was a documentary made by the Barr Foundation, an advocacy group for amputees. Anthony Barr, the foundation's president and a fellow amputee—he lost his foot—narrated the film that described the Ertl procedure. Tragically, Anthony's father, William, was also an amputee, having lost a leg at the mid-thigh. Like me, William Barr's thigh muscles atrophied and retreated from the femur, leaving the nerves and bone unprotected against the constant shock of the prosthetic limb. "For eight years, he too suffered unbearable pain and was told that severing the sciatic nerve was the only solution," Anthony Barr states on the Barr Foundation website. In a 2005 interview for my book, Anthony Barr said that his father's pain was so intense that he considered suicide. "However, in 1979, he [underwent] the Ertl procedure as a 'reconstruction procedure' for his residual limb and was able to live many years with pain-free mobility."

For those who have suffered an amputation at the thigh, as I had, the Ertl procedure involves several complex steps. Excess nerves and any neuromas are removed from the residual limb and arteries and veins are separated. Tiny bits of bone fragments from the upper femur are removed and then transplanted to cover the opening at the bottom of the femur and create a protective bone flap. Finally, the muscles of the thigh are pulled down to cover the bottom of the femur, thus creating a thick padding at the base of the residual limb.

The procedure was invented in 1920 by Dr. Ertl's grandfather, Janos Ertl, Sr., MD. It was now being performed and taught all over the world by Janos's two grandson's, Janika, also known as Jan, and William, a resident at the University of Oklahoma Health Sciences Center.

The Barr Foundation video showed Dr. Jan Ertl performing the operation and then being interviewed afterwards. At every step, Dr. Ertl seemed relaxed and immensely capable. He had performed thousands of these surgeries, Tony Barr reported, and had a greater than 96 percent success rate with the surgery.

I watched the video with my sister Liz, who, at the end of the documentary, said, "He really looks like he knows what he's doing. If I were you, I'd have that procedure done, and I'd have him do it." In an instant, I knew Liz was right.

That did not mean that I was ready to say yes, however. Even though I was in tremendous pain, this was still considered elective surgery, which meant that I would have to take complete responsibility for it if something went wrong. Besides, I had had too much experience with doctors not to be leery. I wasn't ready to trust yet, nor was I ready to make peace with medicine. I need more information. I need to meet Dr. Ertl.

I left a message with Dr. Ertl's office in Sacramento telling him that I was considering reconstructive surgery and that I would like to meet with him. I spoke with him a few weeks later and he told me he would be in Atlanta on March 5 for a medical conference and he asked if we could meet there. I told him that my husband and I would be there. Despite the short, three-day notice, Tom and I made hasty arrangements and on the 5th were waiting in the large foyer of a hotel in Atlanta waiting for Dr. Ertl to emerge from his medical conference.

I liked him the moment I met him. As he approached, I noticed that he had a big, relaxed stride that seemed to radiate a certain comfort he had with himself. His face was friendly and warm. We stepped into an empty conference room and he sat down opposite me and said, "Okay, let's have a look at it."

I was wearing a skirt that I pulled up high enough to expose my residual limb. When he reached toward my leg, I retreated and asked him to be careful. "Any little touch can set off shock-like pains," I told him. He nodded and then gently examined my leg. He was calm and confident. As Tom would say later, "He reminded me of a Chuck Yeager type—you know, the kind of guy that if the engine cuts out at 40,000 feet, he's okay with it. He just tells his passengers not to worry, 'We're all going to be fine.'"

I had already learned that he was in demand all over the world. The Navy had adopted the procedure for its own amputees and he was teaching it in Russia, China, India, and many other countries.

After considering how much pain I was in, Dr. Ertl suggested that I have an MRI done on my leg to determine if a neuroma was the cause. I made a mental note to have the test done as soon as I got home.

"Okay, when can we do it?" he asked. He directed the question to me, but I could tell it was also a rhetorical question that he was asking himself. Suddenly, he brightened. "What about April 2?" he said. "That's a Saturday. The operating room is quiet on Saturdays." I could tell that this man loved his work by his attitude and quiet enthusiasm.

"I can't believe I'm even considering this operation," I said to him.

"That's how most amputees feel," he said. "You have to remember how you feel now so that you can tell other amputees how you felt before you had it done." He was confident that my surgery would be a success.

His confidence was infectious, but it was more than his confidence that swayed me. I felt intuitively that he was competent and that I would be safe with him.

"Do you have a list of patients whom I can call to hear about their experiences with the surgery?" I asked him. He gave me a couple of names and said his secretary would provide the contact information.

By the time we left Atlanta, my soul was saying yes, but my rational mind was still afraid and holding back. Once I got home, I arranged to talk to one of Dr. Ertl's former patients, a man named Chad Thompson. Chad's story was very much like my own. His residual leg had atrophied and, consequently, he had ongoing problems getting a prosthesis to fit. He also suffered intense and chronic pain. But after he had the Ertl reconstruction, his life was changed. "I nearly cried when I took off the bandages," he told me. His residual limb literally had been rebuilt. The stump now had plenty of padding and support against the impact of the prosthetic device. When he put on his prosthesis, he was free from pain, and has been ever since.

I hung up the phone, took pad and pencil in hand, and considered all that I had heard and experienced about the Ertl procedure. On the pad, I wrote, "The Barr Video." It was very persuasive, I felt. I put a check next to it to indicate its positive effect on me. Next, I wrote Dr. Ertl's name. He was completely authentic, sincere, and convincing. Another check. After that, I wrote Chad Thompson. His greatest hopes for the surgery had been realized. Check. Inside, I could feel my fears giving way. It was as if doors inside my heart were starting to open. Out of my heart came some energy, or enthusiasm, that was pushing me toward yes.

There was something still holding me back, however. What else did I need? I asked myself. The answer came immediately.

That night, we had to have a chance to be alone to talk. "I need you to support me if I'm going to have this operation", I told Tom. "I can't do it without your help", I said.

Tom looked away from me and into the middle distance. I could tell that he was looking inside himself. And then he looked back at me and said, "Whatever you want or need, I'll be there."

"I need to get to Sacramento at least a few days before the surgery," I said. "I can't arrive on Friday and have the surgery on Saturday. I've got to have macrobiotic food while we're there, so we'll have to be able to cook. I'm going to need your help the entire time. And I'll need to stay in Sacramento a few days after the surgery just to make sure everything is all right and that I'm healing properly."

"Okay," he said. "We can do all of that."

Tom and I arranged to leave for Sacramento on March 30th. I'd have the operation on April 2, and we'd stay in Sacramento until the 12th, when we planned to return home.

We still had a couple of weeks left before we went to California, and there was still a lot to do. First among them was to have an MRI performed. To expedite the process, I went to my orthopedic doctor in Portland, Maine and told him of my plan asking him to write a prescription for an MRI, as I needed to bring the results with me to Sacramento.

When I returned to Maine after the surgery, I followed up with my orthopedic doctor to show him my leg. Dr. Roma was circumspect. "I'm really impressed with what I saw on the MRI," he said to me.

I wasn't sure what he meant because I hadn't seen the MRI. "Oh, you think I have good bone density," I asked?

"No," he said. "I'm really impressed how large the neuroma was."

We looked at each other. I assumed that this was his way of acknowledging that my suspicions had been correct, and that I must have been in a lot of pain.

AN ANGEL NAMED PEGGY ○ Even though I had come to accept the necessity of the surgery, I was still deeply afraid. I felt as if I were bobbing up and down in the middle of the ocean, lost and adrift, a victim of currents that I could not control. I had no anchor and no way to navigate the flow of events that was about to unfold.

One afternoon as I sat on my couch meditating, I stopped and glanced over at my book shelves where my attention was drawn to one book. *Prepare for Surgery, Heal Faster: A Guide to Mind-Body Techniques*, by Peggy Huddleston. On the shelf next to the book was a cassette tape that was meant to accompany the book. I flipped through the pages. The book was written to help people facing surgery to take control of the process and create positive thoughts before, during, and after their operations. According to the author, such positive thinking can dramatically improve and speed up the healing process.

Suddenly a memory came back to me. A couple of years before, I sat in the waiting room at Women to Women Medical Center and saw the book on display. I paged through it, liked it, and bought it with the intention of giving it away to someone who might need it. Little did I know at the time that I was buying it for myself.

I started listening to the tape every night as I lay in bed and I would be asleep within ten minutes of turning on the recording. In the past, I had trouble falling asleep because of the discomfort of my leg, and certainly the anxiety of the approaching operation should have given me even greater insomnia, but the tapes deeply relaxed me and quickly put me to sleep.

As I read the book and listened to the tape, I felt more and more in control of the process leading up to my surgery. To direct the immune and healing forces to my leg, I tried to imagine myself fully healed. The image that came to my mind was of me riding a bicycle wearing a yellow shirt. I could not ride a two-wheeled bicycle with a prosthetic leg, of course, but I could experience many of the emotions associated with that experience, such as the physical freedom, fitness, joy, and child-like abandon of bicycle riding. I also pictured myself swinging a golf club and walking to the mail box on my prosthetic leg without any pain. These images gave me real joy that flowed through my body.

I wanted the anesthesiologist to make positive, healing statements to me during surgery, which I hoped would draw him to my cause in a personal way. I realized that we were doing this together, and that we had to connect as people.

Everything was now in place to go forward, and I knew in my heart, mind, and body that I was doing the right thing. Without this surgery, I would spend the rest of my life in pain and on crutches. With it, I would be free of pain. My residual limb would be reconstructed so that it could bear weight and wear the prosthetic leg comfortably and I would be free to live a relatively normal life again.

This was my peace with medicine, I realized. I had found a doctor I trusted who would perform an operation I needed. Despite all the difficulties I had had with doctors, and so many legitimate reasons for fears, I found myself feeling gratitude for medicine. Even more, I felt deep gratitude for the divine power that was leading me now, as it had through every difficult challenge. My faith, which had grown stronger over the years, was like a loving hand holding my own. I was not walking into this mystery alone.

SACRAMENTO ○ As our flight descended over Sacramento, I could see the rice fields below us glistening in the California sun. For someone who ate brown rice every day, it was a reassuring sight. I had to admit, however, that the thought of all these jet fumes falling upon the rice gave me pause and some discomfort. I sighed, "Oh well," and let go of another of modern life's compromises.

We arrived on March 30, 2005, and would not return home until the 12th of April. Our hotel was not far from Kaiser Permanente, where my surgery would be performed. The part of town we were in was nearly devoid of nature. It was all concrete, cars, and highways strewn with fast food restaurants. Tom and I took a suite with a kitchen so that we could cook our meals. I didn't want a room that would look out on the street—it was too noisy—so we got a room in the back, where it was quieter and greener, as the windows looked out on some trees and the swimming pool. I was determined to nurture myself even with the little things.

The flight to Sacramento had been pleasant, especially being with Tom. I had wished that we were going on vacation together, rather than having my leg re-amputated. I reassured myself by saying that if all goes well, I'll be able to walk again without crutches, and Tom and I will go on a real vacation together. Still, we were sharing this journey, a deeply spiritual one for both of us. Major surgery is a great risk, no matter how good the doctor is; I knew the risks and accepted them. Meanwhile, with Tom's support and my faith, I kept my goal in sight.

As soon as we were settled in at the hotel, Tom and I wanted to familiarize ourselves with the city. We had done some research before coming and knew that there was a Whole Foods Grocer and a natural foods cooperative nearby, so the first thing we did was go shopping. We stocked up on the staples—whole grains, vegetables, beans, sea vegetables, fruit and snacks—and then went back to our hotel to cook and eat. I also bought myself a decorative tea cup to use during my hospital stay. It was a small way to nurture and support myself, rather than using the hospital's standard bone-colored, heavy cafeteria-style mugs that are so difficult to hold without using both hands.

As we ate, we talked about my plans to make this hospital experience more personal and comfortable. In the past, when I was being treated for cancer, I went to the hospital as most people do—completely unprepared to take care of myself, or to do whatever I could to make the experience more bearable. For example, hospital pillows, sheets, and blankets are often uncomfortable, and the hospital gowns are needlessly cold and revealing.

So, once Tom and I had finished eating, we found a large department store where I bought an inexpensive polar fleece blanket and a good pillow that I could take with me when I traveled to surgery so that I wouldn't be cold in the operating room.

I also needed a CD player that would play the tape continuously throughout the operation. My surgery would take about three hours, and I wanted to listen to healing music. I used earphones that blocked out exterior noise. I listened to a CD by pianist Tim Janis, called *Across Two Oceans.*

Through it all, Tom was engaged and happy to be with me. In the past, he would have thought my requests tedious. He understood the comfort that I sought, so instead we had fun together in the spirit of adventure.

On the day before the surgery, I met the anesthesiologist at Kaiser. He went over my record and then said, "You're not on any prescription pain medication?"

"No," I said.

"Well, you are in very good health because most amputees that have this type of surgery are usually on strong pain killers prior to surgery, which makes them require more anesthesia. You're in really good shape, which means that we won't have to use as much of the drug during your surgery."

Hearing him acknowledge that I was in good health, in spite of my two bouts with cancer, made me feel proud that I'd come so far in my healing. I felt that he was seeing beyond the chart and was seeing me in my present condition, not basing his observations on my past medical history.

"Thank you," I said, beaming.

This doctor would not be my anesthesiologist, but he would pass on all his impressions to the doctor who would be with me throughout the surgery the following day.

"I have a couple of requests for the anesthesiologist tomorrow, if that's okay?" I asked.

I told him about the words I wanted the doctor to say as I was going under the anesthesia, and that I wanted the statements repeated as the surgery was being completed. He assured me that they would accommodate my requests.

"Thank you," I said gratefully. "I wish you were my anesthesiologist."

The next day, I looked for a massage therapist. I went to the food co-op and searched the business cards tacked to the bulletin board. As I did, a woman approached me and asked if I was in line for the bathroom. "No," I said. "I'm looking at the bulletin board, so go ahead of me." There was a long wait for the bathroom, so we started to chat.

"I'm looking for a massage therapist," I said. "You're not a massage therapist by any chance, are you?" I asked jokingly. "No," she laughed. "But my boyfriend is. And he's really good. He teaches massage at one of the local wellness centers, and he's been practicing for 12 years." She ruffled through her purse and found one of his business cards and handing it to me, encouraged me to call him. I called the number and left a message. Later that night, the massage therapist returned my call and said that, as it happened, he had an appointment the next day in the same vicinity of where Tom and I were staying and that he could see me around 7 p.m. His voice crisp, clear, and full of energy—even after a full-day's work.

Joe Lombard is a very skilled massage therapist and he gave me a wonderful massage as well as Reiki, which is a form of healing touch that channels life energy into the body. Afterwards, I felt completely relaxed. He asked if Tom might want a massage, explaining that it is also good for caretakers to be nurtured. I called into the bedroom, where Tom laid watching television, and said, "Tom, it's your turn." And with that, I went to bed.

RECONSTRUCTION ○ The following day, Saturday, April 2, Tom and I arrived at the hospital as instructed at 6:30 in the morning. The admitting room was bright and airy, and I felt as though I was walking into a coffee shop on a Saturday morning. I didn't feel the same old, familiar uneasiness of previous surgeries. Next, I was sent upstairs alone to pre-op. We were both surprised that Tom could not accompany me there.

At the elevator, Tom and I said goodbye and gave each other an excited hug and kiss. I smiled and said, "This is it!" Then I was taken into the elevator and upstairs where I was dressed in a hospital gown and prepared for surgery.

The operation was scheduled to begin at 9:00 a.m. I was taken into the operating room on a gurney, wrapped in a sheet with my Polar Fleece blanket and lying comfortably on my pillow. On my johnny I had taped my requests for my doctors to speak to me during the operation. Dr. Ertl noticed the little note, read it, and responded with a kind of open wonder. "Okay," he said.

As the anesthesiologist sat down next to me, I said, "Thank you for being my anesthesiologist and for coming in on a Saturday."

"It's my pleasure," he said, perhaps a little surprised that I would say anything to him. I immediately had a very good feeling about what was about to take place and was soon asleep.

While the surgery took place, Tom went back to the hotel, changed his clothes, and went for a five-mile run on a bike path that ran along the American River. The day was cloudy, but the sun peaked out every so often. Tom was a little apprehensive, but only because he had no control over the events and wanted them to go well. "As I ran along the river, I thought about Meg in the operating room," Tom said later, "and I felt that the surgery would be a success."

Tom had a strong sense of how different this operation was from my previous surgeries. "When Meg had her other operations, there was a lot of fear. When she had her leg amputated, I realized that life would never be the same again, and I wasn't sure how we were going to cope with it. When she had her breast surgery I wondered whether she would still be alive a year later. But this operation was different. I knew that it was the right decision so that Meg could get refitted for a prosthetic leg and be able to resume her active life."

Tom got back to the hospital and waited for me to come out of surgery. At about noon, he was told that I was in the recovery room and doing fine. At about 12:30 p.m., he went out to the Whole

Foods Grocer, had lunch, and returned just after 1 p.m. A nurse approached him and said that he could go upstairs to my room and see me.

"When I got to Meg's room, I saw that the room was very crowded. Two other patients were in the room, with Meg in the middle bed. All three were separated by curtains. I went over to her and gave her a kiss, and she opened her eyes briefly and recognized me. She was very groggy and I could tell that she was in a great deal of pain. I marveled at her courage and determination. It was very tough to watch her in such pain and feel helpless to do anything about it. Occasionally my eyes would well up with tears and I would think, "Why does she have to go through this suffering and I escape it?"

NO WAY OUT BUT THROUGH ○   The first sound that I heard was my own voice moaning. I wanted to scream, but my life force was still so weak that all I could manage was a faint murmur. During the operation, Dr. Ertl had cut the bottom of my limb and pulled the skin back like a sleeve, thus exposing blood, muscle, nerves, and bone. He removed the neuroma and nonessential nerve tissue, reconstructed the bone and muscle padding at the base of the limb, and then sewed the leg back up. As I began to regain consciousness, the pain from the surgery felt similar to barbed wire wrapped around my leg. I opened my eyes and saw Tom and he bent over and kissed me and told me that he loved me. But the morphine took effect and I quickly fell back to sleep.

During the night, I vaguely remember a Hispanic man and woman entering my darkened room. I didn't know if they were nurses from another floor, but one stood on my left and the other on my right. The man kindly said, "Don't worry, Chica, you have Dr. Ertl and he's the best. He'll take care of you." I could feel the caring and love coming from both of them; even though I don't believe the woman spoke.

Later that night, I woke up in pain. I heard a male nurse, Patrick, come to my bed and respond to my pleas for pain medication with anger.

"You're not pressing the button," he scolded me. "You wouldn't be in so much pain if you pressed that button and medicated yourself."

Still bound by the fog, I asked, What button? Did I form the words? Did my voice find the power to carry them to his ear?

"This button," he said, now thoroughly impatient with me. With that, he took a chord that hung by the side of my bed and threaded it under my hospital bracelet. My hands clumsily grasped for the control. "Okay, so now you have it. Airy fairy," he said as he headed toward the door.

I suddenly sprung into consciousness as though resurrected from the dead and in a deep and commanding voice replied, "Don't you talk to me rudely like that." I perceived his shock and embarrassment at my response. He immediately started backpedaling and stammered, "What did I say that was rude?" Unable to reiterate his words, I snapped, "It was your tone."

Knowing he behaved in an unprofessional manner, he sheepishly made his exit. Meanwhile I lay awake for what felt like a long period of time thinking about what had transpired and struggled to monitor the location of my control so that I could self-administer the drug. I was aware that I didn't want to lose sight of the control and have to ask Patrick for assistance again.

When I woke up early the next morning, I opened my eyes and saw Tom sitting on the left of my bed. He looked at me with love and concern. Tom was always at my bedside, and he would sit in the chair next to me and read, or work on his Blackberry. I felt so much gratitude for his presence as I drifted in and out of sleep for the first four days of my hospital stay.

On Sunday night, I ate a few bites of watermelon while still in a groggy fog. I soon threw up the little I had eaten and then went back to sleep. On Tuesday evening, I ate a few bites of grain and some well-cooked vegetables, chewing them while still half asleep.

On Wednesday morning, I awoke to find Tom standing by my bedside with breakfast. He had made breakfast, lunch, and dinner everyday on the chance that I might wake up and need something to eat. He arrived at 7:30 in the morning each day and didn't leave until 10 or 11 p.m. each night.

When I finally did fully awaken on Wednesday, I was ravenous. Tom had made oatmeal with fruit and two or three different vegetables, all well-cooked so that I could easily digest them. He had also brought a thermos of kukicha tea, a Japanese twig tea that is very soothing and alkalizing— my favorite. I was so pleased to see the silver thermos, as he poured the tea into the porcelain cup we had bought at the health food store.

Before the surgery, I had asked Tom to give my leg palm healing, a form of laying on of hands. This is done by placing your hands over an injured or ill part of the body and then visualizing God's energy flowing through you and into the person you are trying to heal. It is a kind of meditation. Tom was slightly embarrassed, but knew that it was something small that he could do to help me. And whenever he did it, Dr. Ertl came walking into the room, as if on cue, and saw Tom reverently placing his hands over my leg. Dr. Ertl never said anything, but what a strange sight it must have been. "How embarrassing," Tom told me later.

"Thank you, Tom, for your love and support," I told him.

Thanks to Tom, we had become very self-sufficient in the hospital. When a nurse came into the room and said that he would bathe me, I would say, "No, Tom will do that." He helped me to the bathroom, got whatever I needed, and provided three beautiful and life-sustaining meals each day. The nurses were all curious and amazed by the food Tom prepared. One commented "We should all be eating that way," as she curiously eyed my oatmeal, broccoli, and carrots. I felt that I was recovering quickly and on April 8, I was discharged from the hospital. A young, attractive male nurse was in my room filling out my discharge papers and checking my ID bracelet. "Is that your age…47? You look ten years younger than that," he said with real sincerity. This made my day! Outside, I was greeted by the sun.

We returned to our hotel room, where I spent the next four days recuperating and making sure that no complications arose. The days in our hotel were soft, slow, and sweet. I slept a lot and did post-operative exercises to encourage the healing process. Tom made our meals, made us tea, as we talked for hours. He even read to me from *Ordinary Life* by Elizabeth Berg, a book of short stories. One story in particular, about the discontent between a husband and wife and their conflicting emotions and viewpoints was a comical and hilarious tale, and a great antidote. He couldn't have chosen a more amusing story to share with me.

Because the days gave us such an opportunity to be together, I was able to see just how much Tom and I had changed. I thought about how our marriage had shown signs of healing over the past few months. After both of my previous surgeries, Tom went to work every day leading up to the operation, and then went back to work immediately after it. He was able to do that because both of our mothers took care of me. Now, our children were much older, he had more flexibility at work, and he was able to be with me, both physically and spiritually, and I cherished the time we had together. There was so much more joy in the experience, which had to help my healing process. But even the little things revealed how much our relationship had evolved.

A few days before we left for home, I told Tom that I had had an intuition that we would have trouble making our connecting flight in Chicago. There was only a 45 minute lay-over between our arrival in Chicago and our departure for Portland. "Tom, I'll need a sleeping bag in case I need to lie down in the airport,' I said.

"Sure," he replied. Then he commented that I might be right. Tom knew O'Hare airport well and realized that our arrival gate was a significant distance from the gate for our departure. Tom took my request seriously and made sure I had what I needed in case my concerns materialized.

During the last couple of days in the hotel, I practiced sitting up and walking a bit on my crutches, because that's what I would have to do during the long flights home. On April 11, I saw Dr. Ertl, who examined my leg and pronounced me well-along in the healing process. He gave me a big hug and told me that I'd be fine and was ready to go home. I was touched by the hug he gave me, and asked Tom if he wasn't surprised by the gesture. "Everyone loves you, Meg," Tom said.

The following day, we took off from Sacramento to Chicago, hoping to make our connecting flight to Portland. In Chicago, we landed at Gate C23 and had to hurry to Gate F4, one of the longest distances between gates at O'Hare. One of the attendants placed me in a wheelchair and we hurried to the gate. When we finally arrived, the flight had already boarded and the doors were shut. We were stranded. There was nothing to do but go to customer service to arrange another flight, but when we got to the customer service area, there were already long lines of people.

We joined the end of the line and waited. Each person's problem seemed to take forever to resolve. We'd be on this line for hours, I realized. Since early that morning, I had been sitting up for more than six hours. I had to raise my leg to keep the blood from putting pressure on the surgical wound. I knew that I couldn't go on like this. I had to lie down. I wheeled myself out of line and over to the side of the hallway, where I considered lying down.

From near the glass walls, I looked back at Tom. He stood in line and telephoned the airline on his cell phone. Slung over his shoulders were both of our backpacks and the mini sleeping bag I had insisted on taking with us. In one hand, he held another bag that we didn't check, and in the other the cell phone. His shoulders were slightly stooped under all that weight, but he was oblivious to the burden, as he concentrated on getting us a flight. At that moment, he looked like he was carrying the weight of the world, but gave no thought to himself. The image was a metaphor for our lives. I saw his vulnerability, and yet he was acting with such strength and courage. My heart opened. I felt so much love that I wanted to cry. After 23 years of marriage, and all that we had been through, all I could feel was love and gratitude for this man.

On the phone, Tom worked out the arrangements for a new flight, which would not leave for several more hours. I felt the need to put my leg up. Tom and I decided to buy a membership to the United Air Lines Red Carpet Club, not a problem since Tom is a frequent flyer. Tom arranged the furniture so that I could sit back in my chair while elevating my leg on another chair. When I was completely comfortable, he sat down next to me. I took his arm and held him close, resting my head on his shoulder.

"You are heroic," I said. Tom smiled at me.

"Thank you for everything," I said, "for dropping the demands of your job, for coming to California with me, for cooking, for taking care of me, and for all the love you have given me. Thank you for the life we've had together."

Tom kissed me and said, "I love you."

A NEW LIFE ○ At home, I took off the bandages and saw that my leg was beautiful. Miraculously, after 15 years of wear and atrophy, my leg had been reconstructed so that I could wear a prosthesis without pain. In the weeks and months ahead, I hoped that I could be fitted properly with a prosthesis and look forward to walking, strolling through my neighborhood, going grocery shopping, and maybe even taking up golf again.

One day that spring, while cutting vegetables by the open window of my kitchen, I suddenly had a strange and surprising thought. I had cancer to thank, and all the trials and tribulations that accompanied it, for helping me banish my fears, find my voice and mission, and find—really find—happiness.

Given the chance, my life might have unfolded in a very predictable way, without me ever realizing all that I might have missed. But fate stepped in and I was diagnosed with cancer, which in turn led me to macrobiotics and a new world of hope, adventure, and endless possibilities. This new world helped restore the love between Tom and me—a gift for which I'll always be grateful.

Dealing with cancer ultimately led me to a place in my life where I was able to heal my physical body, as well as my heart and soul. I stand now facing my new and wonderful life—bearing the wounds of a hard-won battle—a stronger, more creative and passionate, and happy woman. And grateful for the gift I've been given.

PHOTO ALBUM

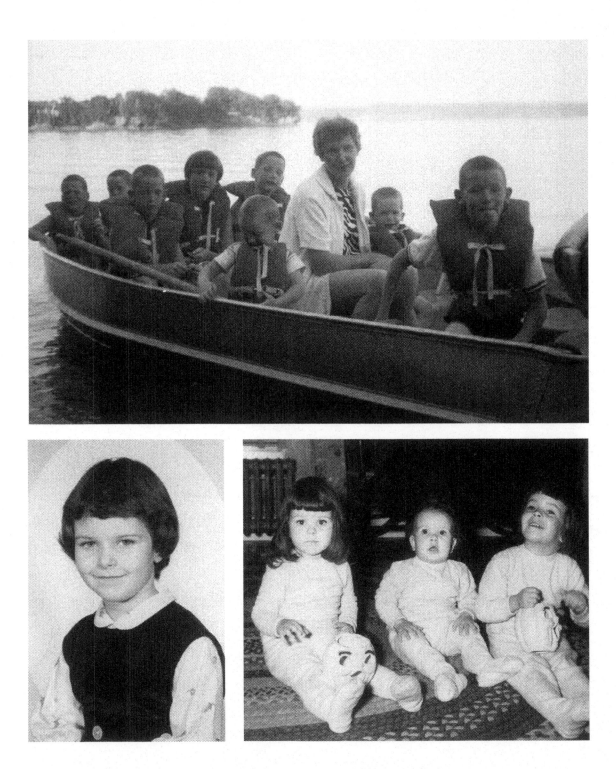

TOP: Tom (far right) at age 11 with his mom and siblings at Lake Champlain, Vermont (1967). **BOTTOM LEFT:** Me at age 7, St. Hyacinth's School, Westbrook, Maine (1965). **BOTTOM RIGHT:** Me (age 2) with sisters Liz (age 1) and Martha (3½) (1959).

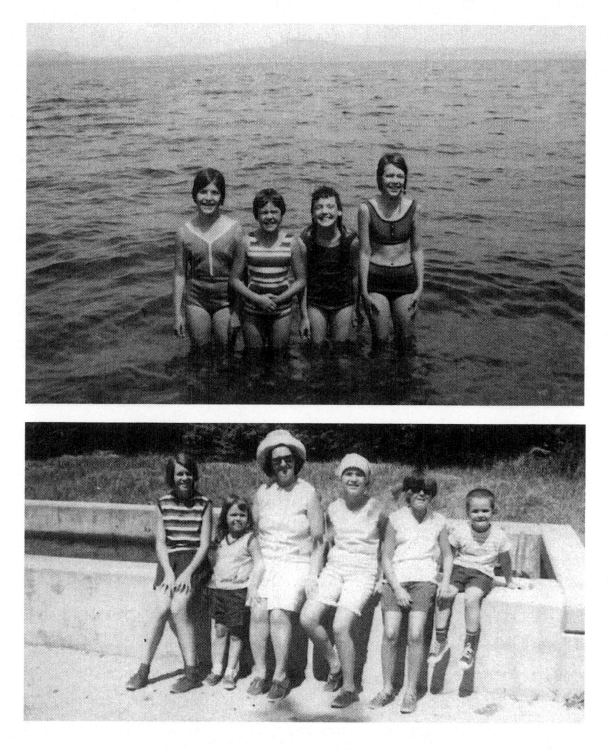

TOP: Me (age 12), Liz, (friend Katie) and Martha at Sebago lake, Maine (1968). **BOTTOM:** My sisters Martha, Ruth, my mom, me, Liz, and my brother Bill at the Fish Hatchery, Gray, Maine (1968).

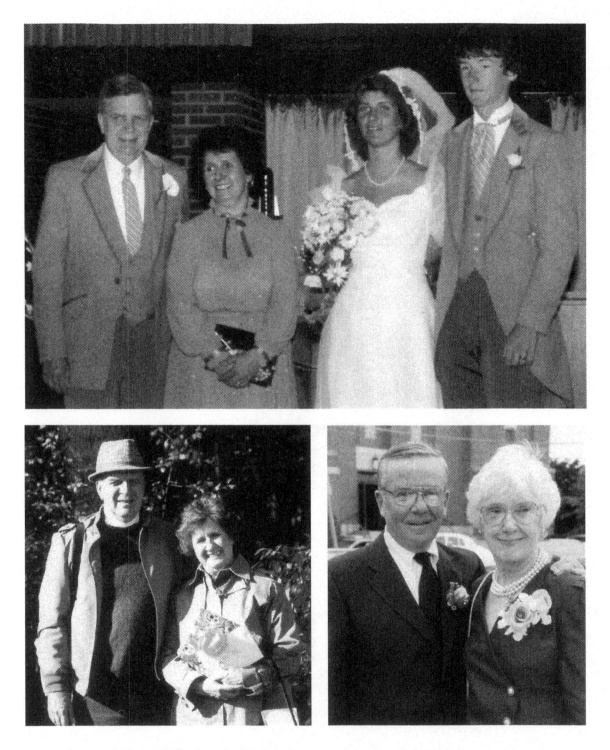

TOP: Our wedding in Westbrook, Maine, August 21, 1982. **BOTTOM LEFT:** My parents Mark and "Wally" DeCoste visiting us in 1987 in Rockland, Mass. **BOTTOM RIGHT:** Tom's parents Charlie and Alice Wolff at Tom's brother's, wedding Long Island, NY, 1993.

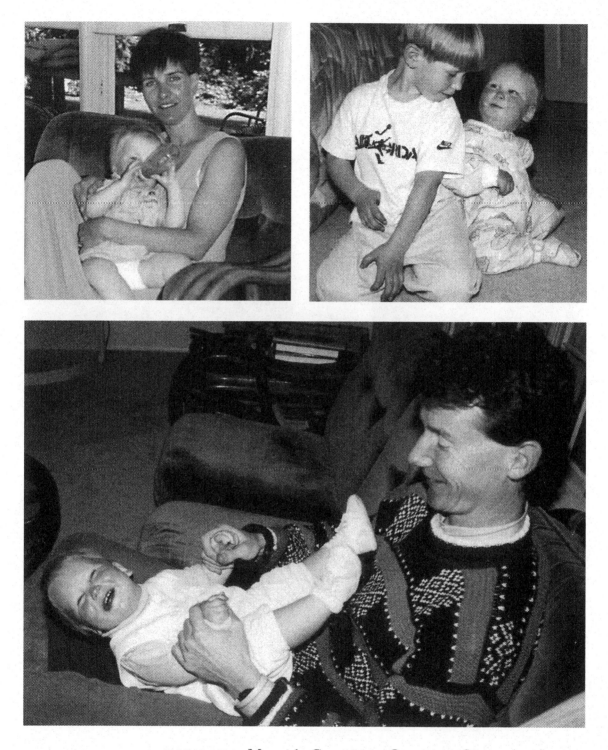

TOP LEFT: Me with Cammie in Oregon in Spring (1991). **TOP RIGHT:** Francis (age 5) with Cammie (age 1) (1991). **BOTTOM:** Tom with Cammie (age 1) (1991).

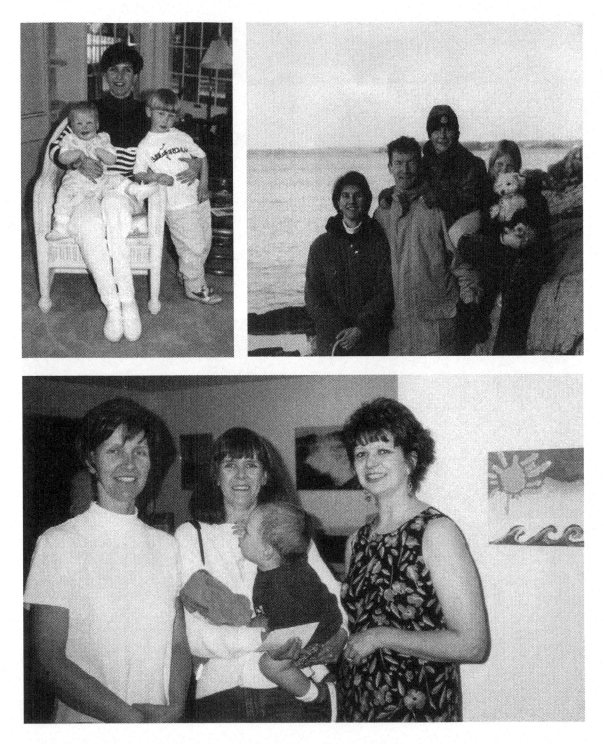

TOP LEFT: Me with Cammie and Francis in February, 1991. **TOP RIGHT:** Me, Tom, Francis (age 12), Cammie (age 8) and Cuddles, a few days after my diagnosis of breast cancer in 1998. **BOTTOM:** Me (with wig), Liz (with son Stephen) and Ruth in the fall of 1999 when I was finishing chemotherapy.

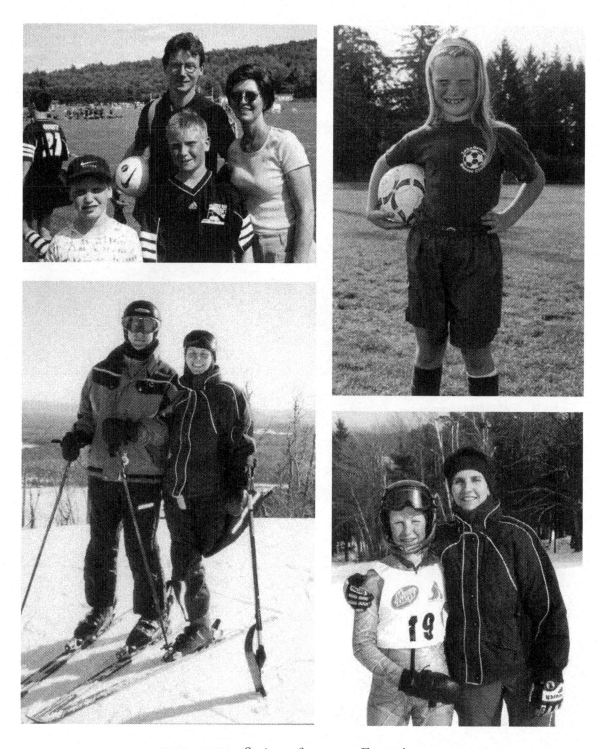

TOP LEFT: Spring of 1999 at Francis' soccer game. **TOP RIGHT:** Cammie's soccer picture in 1995. **BOTTOM LEFT:** Tom and Me (3 track skiing) at Sunday River, Maine (2000), **BOTTOM RIGHT:** Cammie (age 10) and Me at a ski race (2000).

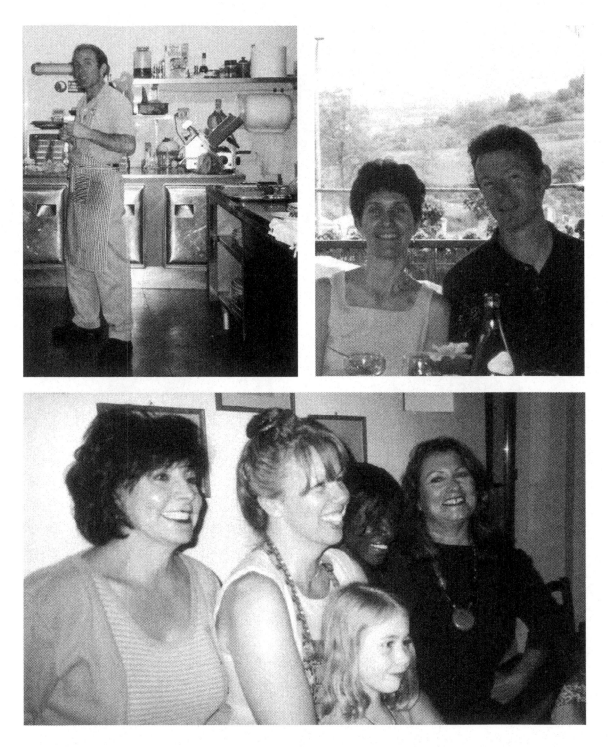

TOP LEFT: Warren Kramer (my macrobiotic counselor) in Italy, in May 2001, with Christina Pirello's MacroTour. **TOP RIGHT:** Me and Tom on Christina's Italy trip (2001). **BOTTOM:** Christina Pirello (second to the left) on her MacroTour in Italy.

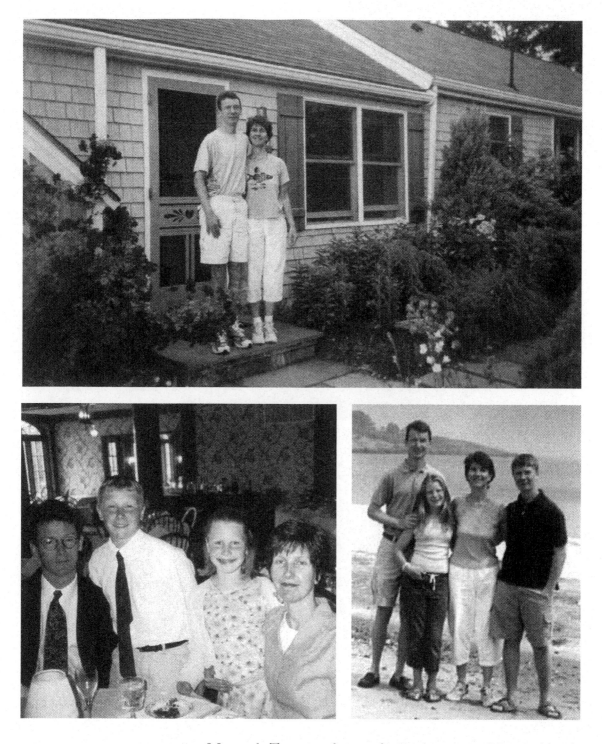

TOP: Me and Tom in front of our home in Maine (2002). **BOTTOM LEFT:** My family in the spring of 1999, while I was undergoing chemo. **BOTTOM RIGHT:** Tom, Cammie (age 12), Me, Francis (age 16) on the beach in back of our house.

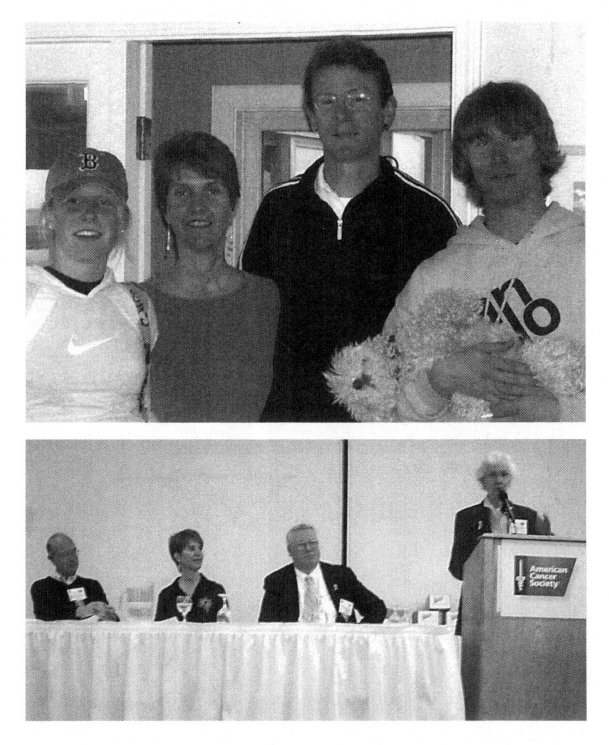

TOP: Cammie (age 14), Me, Tom, Francis (age 18) and our dog Cuddles (2004). **BOTTOM:** Me (middle) seated on the survivor panel of the Living With Cancer Conference in May 2005.

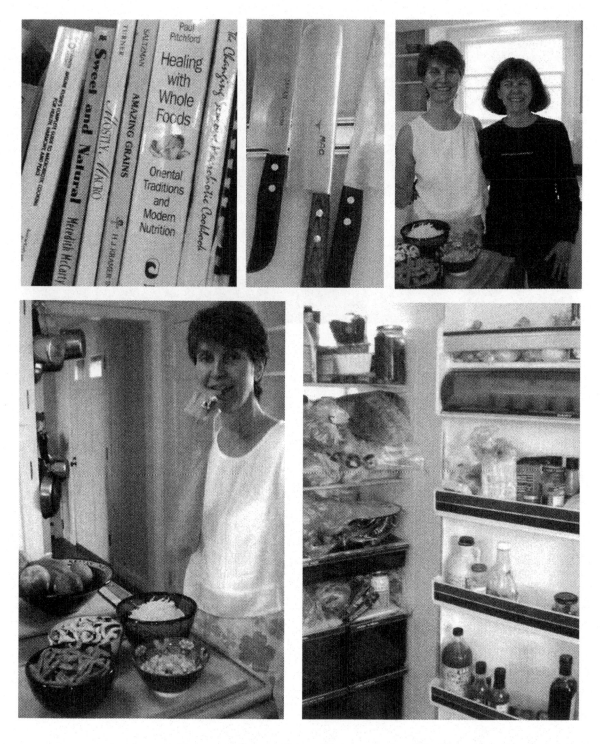

TOP LEFT: Some of the titles on my bookshelf. **TOP MIDDLE:** My knives—this type of knife is the most important tool in macrobiotic cooking. **TOP RIGHT:** Me and Liz in my kitchen. **BOTTOM LEFT:** Me sampling the veggies. **BOTTOM RIGHT:** A sneak peak inside my refrigerator. *All photos on this page taken in 2005 by my niece Kate Delaney for a school project.*

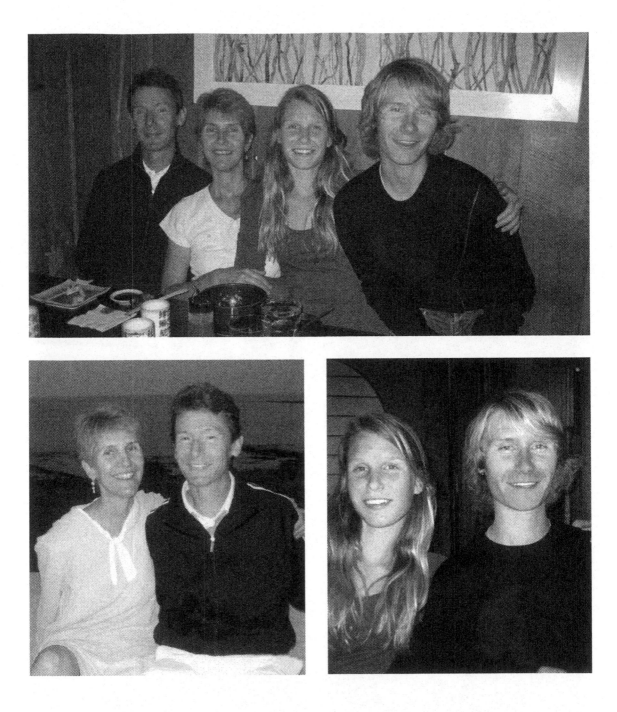

TOP : Tom, Me, Cammie and Francis celebrating Francis' 20th birthday at Sapporo Restaurant in Portland Maine, August 2006 **BOTTOM RIGHT:** Tom and Me, August 2006 **BOTTOM LEFT:** Cammie and Francis, August 2006

PART TWO

A dietary and lifestyle approach to cancer.

After I was diagnosed with bone cancer, and later with breast cancer, I asked my doctors if there was any link between cancer and diet. All but two dismissed the idea, and a few thought the notion was ridiculous. In fact, scientists have found that certain kinds of diets are clearly linked to an increased risk of cancer. More important, diet can influence how long a person survives after he or she is diagnosed with cancer. Researchers consistently have found that eating a plant-based diet, one that is made up primarily of whole grains, fresh vegetables, beans, and fruit, is associated with longer life in people who have been diagnosed with cancer, especially with breast cancer.

There are seven reasons why a diet such as the macrobiotic regimen can help people with cancer, and especially women with breast cancer. The macrobiotic diet helps because it is:

1. Extremely low in fat and cholesterol.
2. Low in calories.
3. Advocates the elimination of milk products.
4. Rich in fiber.
5. Rich in plant-based compounds that boost the immune and cancer-fighting forces in the body.
6. Contains many specialty foods, such as miso and other soy foods, shiitake mushrooms, and sea vegetables, all of which directly fight cancer.
7. Stresses organic foods and the elimination of synthetic pesticides, fertilizers, and herbicides, all of which can contribute to breast cancer.

Once a woman contracts breast cancer, she faces many important questions, but none more important than this one: Do women who eat a diet made up largely of plant foods live longer? The answer is an unequivocal yes.

I

LOWER THE FAT AND ANIMAL FOOD CONTENT OF YOUR DIET AND LIVE LONGER ○ Women with breast cancer who eat a plant-based diet tend to live longer than those who eat more animal foods. This is just one of the findings that have come out of the research of Dr. James Hebert and his colleagues at the University of Massachusetts (UMASS) Medical School. Hebert showed that diet greatly influences the chances that a breast cancer will recur, or reappear, after it has been forced into remission after treatment. When a cancer recurs, it is much more difficult to control, and therefore much more dangerous.

Hebert, whose study was published in the medical journal, *Breast Cancer Research and Treatment* (September, 1998) found that consumption of foods high in fat, including dairy products, was associated with shorter survival among women with breast cancer. Butter, beef, liver, and bacon are especially dangerous, Hebert found. Pre-menopausal women with breast cancer, who regularly ate butter, margarine, and lard, had a 67 percent greater chance of cancer recurrence than women who abstained from these foods. Women who ate beef, liver, and bacon had a much higher rate of recurrence of breast cancer than women who abstained from these foods.

On the other hand, women who ate more plant foods tended to live longer. Simply eating more vegetables each day was associated with lower rates of recurrence, Hebert found. The women who ate the most vegetables had the fewest recurrences and lived the longest, while those who ate the fewest had the shortest survival on average. The UMASS scientists found that each additional serving of vegetables consumed each day translated into a 53 percent *reduction* in risk of recurrence.

Vegetables and fruits rich in vitamin C greatly increase the chances that a woman with breast cancer will live longer. Post-menopausal women who ate broccoli, collard greens, kale, and citrus fruits lived longer than women who abstained from these foods. Each additional 100 mg. of vitamin C—over the amount eaten from the standard diet—reduced the risk of recurrence by 43 percent. (You will recall that I had vitamin C injections during my chemotherapy.)

Another study followed 678 women with breast cancer. All had similar degrees of illness; all had undergone similar forms of treatment; and all had been estimated to have a 90-percent chance of surviving five years. The scientists found, however, that those women who ate high fat diets had the shortest survival time. The scientists calculated that for every five percent increase in saturated fat from animal sources, the risk of dying increased by 50 percent.

That same study, published in a 1994 issue of the *Journal of the National Cancer Institute*, found that those women who had higher intakes of plant foods rich in vitamin C and beta carotene—the vegetable source of vitamin A—from plant sources experienced a 50 percent reduction in the risk of dying. Overall, women who ate more of the foods rich in these vitamins lived longer.

2

REDUCE EXCESS CALORIES TO INCREASE YOUR CHANCES OF RECOVERY ○ Another UMASS study found that the number of calories a woman with breast cancer eats—especially calories from fatty animal foods—can also determine how long she lives. A study published in the *Journal of Breast Cancer Research and Treatment* (February 1999) found that women with breast cancer who ate an additional 1000 calories above their optimal calorie levels experienced an 84 percent increase in the risk of recurrence.

It's actually easy to get an additional 1000 calories simply by eating a few processed foods each day. Those women who did experienced much higher rates or recurrence. On the other hand, whole foods—such as whole grains, fresh vegetables, beans, and fruit—are low in calories. A diet made up mostly of these foods is a low-calorie diet.

One of the reasons calorie intake is so important is because the higher the calories, the higher the insulin levels and the greater the weight gain. Insulin is the hormone produced by your pancreas to make blood sugar available to your cells. Your cells use blood sugar as their primary fuel. The more processed foods you eat, the higher your insulin levels. And the higher your insulin levels, the greater your risk of recurrence of cancer. Many scientists now believe that this combination—high calorie diet, overweight, and high insulin, now referred to as syndrome X—is the underlying cause of much of the breast cancer we see today.

Being overweight is poisonous to women, especially women with breast cancer. National Institutes of Health researchers have shown that weight loss, especially when it occurs in women in mid-life, significantly reduces their risk of breast cancer. Dr. Regina Ziegler and her co-workers followed 1,563 women for more than two decades. The scientists, whose study was published in the *Journal of the National Cancer Institute* (1996: 88, 650-660), found that women who had shed excess weight in their 40s and 50s cut their risk of getting breast cancer in half.

Women with breast cancer must understand that weight can determine how long they live. Obesity, very often a direct result of dietary fat intake, increases the risk of dying of breast cancer. The Iowa Women's Health Study, which examined 698 postmenopausal women with breast cancer, found that overweight women are nearly twice as likely to die of breast cancer than lean women. Not surprisingly, the researchers also found that women with the highest dietary fat intake also have twice the risk of dying of breast cancer.

The reason weight loss plays such an important role, of course, is that it dramatically affects both men and women's hormone levels. In women, the hormone in question is estrogen, which can act like a trigger for breast and other cancers. The higher the estrogen levels, the greater your risk of cancer. And the higher your weight, and the fat content of your diet, the more estrogen in your body.

ESTROGEN AND BREAST CANCER ◦ Estrogen helps develop and sustain the health of the hormone sensitive organs, namely the ovaries, uterus, and breasts. Most of a woman's estrogen is produced by her ovaries, at least up until menopause. At menopause, the ovaries significantly reduce their estrogen production. But another major source of estrogen is fat cells. The larger and more numerous the fat cells, the more estrogen a woman's body produces.

Each month, estrogen surges in a woman's body to produce her menstrual cycle. During that time, the uterus fills with blood and the breasts become inflamed and sensitive. When excess estrogen is produced by the body, these organs become overstimulated. The periods can be come excessively heavy and the breasts swollen, tender, and painful.

Estrogen can act like growth hormone, triggering the over-production of tissue inside the breast and uterus. The more estrogen you have, the more enflamed your breast tissue becomes, and the more tissue you produce within the breast itself. This combination of inflammation and excess tissue can combine to block milk ducts, as well as blood and lymph vessels within the breast, causing waste products to stagnate within the breast. This can create the conditions for fibrocystic breasts and, eventually, breast cancer.

Diets rich in fat and animal proteins are associated with a wide array of hormone-related disorders. For example, young women on high-fat diets experience their first periods much sooner than women on plant-based diets. Teenage British girls, whose diets provide an average of 43 percent calories from fat, get their first period at an average age of 13. Chinese girls, on the other hand, eat diets made up largely of plant foods—they consume only 15 percent total calories in fat—and on average get their periods at age 17.

As you may know, researchers have found that women who got their periods early in life have a significantly increased risk of contracting breast cancer later in life. Women who eat high-fat diets also experience more abnormal uterine bleeding and heavy periods. This occurs because the uterus is overstimulated by high estrogen, causing more blood to accumulate and much more problematic periods, often characterized by blood clots, heavy bleeding, and pain.

Women on high fat diets have also been shown to experience much more premenstrual syndrome, especially emotional distress, breast swelling, bloating, and fatigue.

Further, high fat diets are associated with a much higher incidence of fibrocystic breast disease. Higher than normal estrogen levels cause inflammation, which produces more cysts, scaring, and tumors.

DIETARY FAT, BACTERIA, AND ESTROGEN ○ To keep estrogen levels down, and thus prevent the hormone from accumulating within tissues, the body allows estrogen to circulate through the system only once. This is accomplished by the liver, which places a chemical compound that attaches to the estrogen and prevents it from being reabsorbed by the small intestine. Unfortunately, women who eat high fat diets promote the growth of bacteria in their colon stripping this compound from the estrogen molecule, thus allowing it to be reabsorbed into the blood stream. Thus, people on high fat diets are not only recirculating the same quantity of estrogens over and over, but they are also producing new estrogen. That new estrogen is coming from their ovaries, as well as from their fat cells. The result is dramatically higher estrogen levels in a woman's body.

These same bacteria that uncouple the estrogen from its non-absorbable compound also produce estrogen-like chemicals themselves that add to the estrogen load in a woman's body.

Finally, women who have high estrogen levels, brought on by high-fat diets, experience menopause later in life and also have higher rates of breast cancer. The reason, scientists speculate, is because the breasts are being overstimulated over longer periods of time, thus increasing the likelihood of triggering a cancer within the breast tissue.

One of the many benefits of a macrobiotic diet is the presence of health-promoting fermented foods, such as miso, tamari, shoyu, tempeh, sauerkraut, and pickles. These foods replenish the intestinal tract with friendly bacteria that release oxygen and promote healthy digestion and assimilation. These same foods also create a more alkaline blood and intestinal environment, both of which make the body highly resistant to disease. The presence of fermented foods in the diet is also important because so many of us have taken antibiotics that destroy friendly flora and create a more acidic intestinal condition, which forms the basis for disease.

3

AVOID MILK PRODUCTS TO PROTECT YOUR BREASTS AND REPRODUCTIVE ORGANS ○
Dairy products—including milk, cheese, and yogurt—can injure your health in a wide array of ways. Much of the dairy people eat today is tainted with trace levels of hormone and antibiotics that have been injected into the animals themselves, and then turn up in their milk. These hormones add to the already existing hormonal imbalance in the body, and thus contribute to breast and ovarian cancers. But there are other reasons to avoid milk products, especially if you want to avoid breast and reproductive cancers.

Milk products are also rich in fat, which increases the estrogen content of your body. But even if you eat organic skim milk, you're still getting substances that increase your risk of cancer.

All milk products, including milk, yogurt, and cheese, cause your blood to contain higher levels of a substance known as insulin-like growth factor (IGF-1), which has been shown to promote the growth of cancers of the breast and prostate. Women with high levels of IGF-1 have been shown to have much higher rates of breast cancer, while men with the highest levels of IGF-1 have four times the rates of prostate cancer, according to a 1998 study published in *Science*.

Dr. Walter Willet, M.D., Ph.D, who is dean of the school of Nutrition at the Harvard Medical School, urges people to avoid milk. In his book, *Eat, Drink, and Be Healthy* (Simon and Schuster, 2000), Dr. Willett, reported the following:

"In nine separate studies, the strongest and most consistent dietary factor linked with prostate cancer was high consumption of milk or dairy products. In the largest of these, the Health Professionals Follow-up Study, men who drank two or more glasses of milk a day were almost twice as likely to develop advanced or metastatic (spreading) prostate cancer as those who didn't drink milk at all."

Milk doesn't just affect the reproductive organs of men, however. A study done in 1989 by Harvard University's Daniel Cramer, M.D. and published in the *Lancet* showed that lactose is transformed in the body to another sugar known as galactose. Cramer showed that when galactose levels exceed a certain threshold in the body, they injure the ovaries and lead to ovarian cancer.

Cramer's work has been corroborated by other researchers, most recent study published in the *American Journal of Clinical Nutrition* (November 2004) that showed that women who consumed four or more dairy products a day suffered significantly increased rates of ovarian cancers.

Milk triggers adverse immune reactions within the body, as well. Often, these reactions can cause immune cells to attack healthy tissues, deforming and destroying healthy cells. This can occur in sensitive children and lead to serious illnesses, including Type I, or childhood diabetes.

In July, 1992, *The New England Journal of Medicine* published a study that showed that cow's milk increased the risk of diabetes in children. The study showed that children produced antibodies in response to proteins in cow's milk, specifically bovine albumin peptide. Scientists speculate that the protein in cow's milk attaches itself to the pancreas. This stimulates the immune system to attack both the proteins and healthy pancreatic tissue. In the process, immune antibodies destroy the insulin-producing beta cells of the pancreas, as well, thus eliminating the ability of the pancreas to produce insulin. This study has since been replicated numerous times.

Diabetes, both children's diabetes, known as Type I, and adult onset, known as Type II, turns up most often in wealthy populations that consume large quantities of dairy products. It's rare in populations, such as Asia and Africa, that do not consume cow's milk. On the other hand, children who are breast-fed have a reduced risk of getting diabetes.

4

TO KEEP YOUR ESTROGEN LEVELS LOW, EAT A HIGH FIBER DIET ○ I mentioned earlier that estrogen is a big promoter of breast cancer, as well as other forms of cancer. Therefore, we want to do all we can to keep our estrogen levels well within the safe ranges. That's where fiber comes in.

Think of fiber as a sponge. It soaks up excess hormone, including estrogen, and helps eliminate it through the feces. Fiber is the reason that vegetarian women who eat lots of plant foods eliminate two to three times more estrogen than non-vegetarians, according to a study published in *The New England Journal of Medicine* (1982).

Another study, reported in the scientific journal, *Nutrition* (1995), showed that a high-fiber, low-fat diet lowered estrogen levels in a group of postmenopausal women by 50 percent. Cutting estrogen levels in half can have an astounding impact on health. Researchers have shown that a 17 percent reduction of estrogen can reduce the risk of breast cancer four to fivefold, according to a report the *Journal of the National Cancer Institute*. Reducing estrogen by 50 percent, in effect, dramatically reduces the inflammatory effects of estrogen and thereby protects breast, uterine, and ovarian tissues.

FIBER: IT KEEPS YOU MOVING • Before I was diagnosed with breast cancer, I consistently suffered from consistent intestinal and bowel disorders. This is no coincidence. Women who are chronically constipated have two to four times more breast disease—such as cysts, lumps, and breast cancer—than women who enjoy good bowel health. One of the reasons, of course, is that healthy women eliminate so much more estrogen through their feces than women who are constipated. Constipation results in recirculating many estrogens.

But constipation also results in high levels of poisons, known as cytotoxins, in your blood stream. Constipation causes these toxins to be reabsorbed through your intestinal tract and then into your lymph and bloodstream. Once in the lymph, they migrate upward toward the clavicle bones, where lymph fluid is sent back into the blood stream and on to the liver, where it is cleansed. But before it gets to the clavicles, located in your shoulders, it passes through your breast tissue, where it can accumulate to create an even more polluted environment in your breasts. Constipation, therefore, can actually add to the toxic load in your breast tissue.

High fiber diets speed intestinal transit time and promote elimination, thus keeping the blood and lymph cleaner—which in turn keeps your breast tissue cleaner.

5

PLANT FOODS ARE RICH IN HEALING COMPOUNDS THAT FIGHT CANCER ○ For the person who is combating a serious illness, the macrobiotic diet is an ideal cancer-fighting diet. It is low in fat, rich in fiber, and abundant in cancer-fighting chemicals.

The diet is composed primarily of whole grains (generally about 40 percent of the diet is grain), fresh vegetables (about 25 percent), beans (about ten percent), and sea vegetables, soups, condiments, and fruit. These vegetables foods are supplemented with fish. As I said earlier, macrobiotic proponents encourage people to eat only organic foods, especially if you are attempting to use the food to overcome a serious illness. These foods, scientists have found, boost the body's healing forces, and directly fight cancer.

Dr. James Carter and his colleagues at the Tulane School of Public Health showed that men with prostate cancer who followed a macrobiotic diet lived longer than men who received standard medical treatment.

In a study published in the *Journal of the American College of Nutrition*, Carter found similar results in men with pancreatic cancer. Those who followed a macrobiotic diet lived substantially longer than those who were treated with standard medical care. Carter followed patients' pancreatic cancer for one year and found that 54.2 percent of those who adopted a macrobiotic diet were still alive one year after diagnosis, while 10 percent of those who underwent only standard medical care were still alive.

Women with lung cancer who ate higher amounts of vegetables and fruits experienced longer survival than those who ate vegetables infrequently, according to a study done by Dr. Marc Goodman of the Cancer Research Center at the University of Hawaii. Consumption of broccoli and other foods rich in vitamin C was consistently associated with longer survival time.

Researchers at the Fred Hutchinson Cancer Research Center in Seattle, Washington, have found that vegetables protect men from prostate cancer. The scientists discovered that men who eat at least three servings of vegetables per day have half the risk of contracting prostate cancer than men who fail to eat those three daily servings, according to a study published in the January 2000 issue of the *Journal of the National Cancer Institute.*.

The vegetables that appear most protective against cancer are the cruciferous variety, namely broccoli, cabbage, collard greens, kale, mustard greens, and watercress. Also included in this family are sauerkraut and cole slaw, both made from cabbage.

"When we compared relative potency, vegetables from the cruciferous family, like broccoli and cabbage, reduced the risk even further," said Dr. Alan Kristal, one of the researchers on the study. The scientists rigorously examined the eating habits of 1,230 men in the Seattle-area between the ages of 40 and 64. Overall vegetable consumption provided strong protection against prostate cancer, but the cruciferous vegetables were the strongest.

"At any given level of total vegetable consumption, as the percent of cruciferous vegetables increased, the prostate cancer risk decreased," Dr. Kristal told Reuters news service.

The cruciferous vegetables contain a substance known as sulforanphane, which promotes detoxification of the blood and tissues and helps to fight cancer. Another is the chemical known as phenethyl isothiocyanate (PEITC), which may inhibit the emergence of lung tumors in animals that have been bred to create cancerous tumors.

PLANTS CONTAIN THE ANTIOXIDANTS ○ The underlying cause of most of the illnesses we face today, including breast cancer, is oxidation, or the breakdown of cells, tissues, and organs. Oxidation is the process that causes iron to rust and apples to turn brown when left out on your counter for too long. In the body, oxidation is caused when healthy cells encounter oxygen-free radicals, which are highly reactive oxygen molecules that kill or deform cells. Free radicals can turn healthy organs into masses of non-functioning scar tissue, causing cirrhosis of the liver, atherosclerosis in the coronary arteries, cataracts in the eyes, and Alzheimer's and Parkinson's disease in the brain. Free radicals can also deform the DNA of your cells, turning healthy cells into malignant cancers.

The antidote to free radicals is antioxidants, which slow down or stop oxidation. Antioxidants protect your cells, tissues, and organs from oxidation, and thus prevent most of the illnesses people suffer form today, such as heart disease, high blood pressure, Alzheimer's, Parkinson's disease, and the common cancers, such as cancer of the breast.

There are literally hundreds, and perhaps thousands of antioxidants, though most of us know the most commonly reported antioxidants, vitamins C, E, and beta carotene. Plant foods are the primary source of all antioxidants.

Without antioxidants, your risk of cancer rises dramatically, according to Bruce Ames, Ph.D., professor of biochemistry and molecular biology at the University of California, Berkeley, and a long-time researcher. Dr. Ames says that people who eat fewer than five servings of antioxidant-rich foods each day experience twice the risk of developing cancer than those who get those five servings.

The body's primary cancer fighter is natural killer cells, which researchers have found are boosted in both number and aggressiveness when you eat antioxidant-rich foods. The Chinese, for example, eat a diet based primarily on grains and vegetables. Their diets are loaded with antioxidants and, not surprisingly, they have low rates of the common cancers, especially breast cancer. Studies have consistently shown that people whose diets are rich in vitamin C have lower rates of breast, colon, and prostate cancers.

Two other groups of chemicals in plant foods are known as carotenoids—the substances that cause your grains, greens, and roots to have color—and phytochemicals, which simply means plant chemicals. Carotenoids are powerful cancer fighters. They include substances you may have heard of such as bioflavonoids, indoles, saponins, and isoflavones.

Studies have shown that bioflavonoids suppress tumor growth, prevent blood clots, and reduce inflammation. Bioflavonoids are found in apples, celery, cherries, cranberries, kale, onions, black and green teas, red wine, parsley, and soybeans.

Scientists continue to be amazed by the crucifer vegetables, which convert cancer-causing estrogens into their more benign forms and thereby prevent breast cancer.

Whole grains and soy products are rich in saponins, which neutralize enzymes in the intestines that cause colon cancer. Sterols, found mostly in vegetables, lower blood cholesterol levels.

The most celebrated group of phytochemicals is isoflavones. These substances, which act as mild estrogens, protect cells from the cancer causing estrogen. They also perform an almost magical feat called anti-angiogenesis, which means, essentially, that isoflavones block blood vessels from attaching to tumors, and thus block the flow of oxygen and nutrients to tumors. Isoflavones also act as antioxidants. Great sources of isoflavones are soy products, whole grains, berries, fruit, vegetables, and flax seeds. The macrobiotic diet is rich in isoflavones, thanks to the presence of soybean products, such as miso, tempeh, tofu, tamari, shoyu, and natto.

6

MACROBIOTIC SPECIALTY FOODS FOR FIGHTING DISEASE ○ The most widely reported isoflavone, of course, is *genistein*, found primarily in fermented soybean products. A study published in the April 1993 *Proceedings of the National Academy of Sciences* showed genistein has a particularly powerful anti-angiogenesis effect. Scientists believe that the great abundance of genistein in diets of Asian women may be one reason why these women do not have the rates of breast cancer women in the West experience, and why Asian women also have much better rates of survival from breast cancer than Western women do.

The primary sources of genistein in the macrobiotic diet are the following:

FERMENTED SOYBEAN PRODUCTS:
Miso is a product made from soybeans that has been aged and fermented in sea salt and a whole grain, such as brown rice, barley, millet, or wheat. The aging process can take anywhere from six months to three years. Miso is used as a base for soup, stews, and sauces. Not only is it rich in isoflavones, but also health-promoting bacteria.

Tempeh. A fermented soybean patty, used in soups, stews, and fried. It is rich in protein, vitamins, minerals, isoflavone, and friendly bacteria.

Tofu. A soybean product that has been pressed to remove some of the fiber and water. It is rich in calcium, protein, isoflavones, and many vitamins and minerals.

Natto. Fermented soybeans used as a condiment on whole grains, vegetables, and noodles.

Shoyu. High quality soy sauce, made from fermented soybeans, and used as the base for soups, stews, and sauces. Low-sodium shoyus are widely available.

Tamari. The liquid runoff from miso production. Tamari often contains a grain, such as brown rice or wheat. Low-sodium tamari is widely available.

Although genistein is most concentrated in soybean products, all beans contain isoflavones.

Researchers now believe that one of the reasons that both Asian and Hispanic women experience such low rates of breast cancer is their high consumption of beans and bean products.

All whole grains, beans, green, yellow, and orange vegetables contain isoflavones. And all the green leafy, orange, red, and yellow vegetables are abundant sources of phytochemicals and carotenoids.

SHIITAKE MUSHROOMS:
Studies at the U.S. National Cancer Institute and the Japanese National Cancer Institute have established the shiitake mushroom as a cancer fighter, an immune booster, and a powerful cholesterol-lowering herb.

The pioneer of shiitake research was Kisaku Mori, Ph.D., who founded the Institute of Mushroom Research in Tokyo. Mori documented the healing effects of shiitake mushrooms and tried to isolate the most active compounds within the mushroom.

One of those compounds, called eritadenine, has been shown by both American and Japanese researchers to dramatically lower blood cholesterol. Studies have shown that three ounces (or 5 or 6 mushrooms) a day can lower blood cholesterol by

12 percent in one week. Other research has suggested that the cholesterol lowering effect of shiitake extract—the concentrated form of the mushroom—may be as much as 25 percent when used over a couple of weeks.

Certain polysaccharides, or long chains of sugars, found in shiitake have been shown to boost immune response. Numerous other immune cells and chemicals to respond more vigorously to a virus, cancer cells, and bacteria after shiitake have been eaten.

In a study published by the U.S. medical journal, *Cancer Research* (1970), scientists reported that six of ten laboratory animals with cancer experienced remission after eating shiitake extract for short periods of time. When the quantities of extract were increased, all ten animals went into remission. Similar findings have been reported by other researchers.

Shiitake has been found to inhibit the attempts of viruses to replicate themselves. Further, scientists at Japan's Yamaguchi University School of Medicine have found that shiitake extract protected cells against the destruction normally caused by HIV infection. The scientists went on to recommend that shiitake be used on conjunction with other HIV and AIDS treatments.

A substances isolated in shiitake called cortinelin has been found to be an effective broad spectrum antibiotic, while the sulfides in shiitake can kill ringworm, fungus, and other skin diseases.

SEA VEGETABLES:

Seaweeds, also known as sea vegetables, are among the most nutritious foods on earth. One hundred grams of nori, which is used to make sushi, contains 28.3 mg. of iron (the RDA is 15 mg. per day); 3,503 mg. of potassium (the RDA is 1,800); 17,800 International Units (IU) of beta carotene (the vegetable source of vitamin A; the RDA is 4,500 mg.); 1.34 of riboflavin B2 (the RDA is 1.7 mg.) and 22.2 mg. of protein (the RDA is 65 mg.). (All nutrient information from the U.S. Department of Agriculture and the Food Composition Table of East Asia.) Nori can be purchased as "sushi nori", which requires no cooking. It comes in flat sheets and is used to wrap around rice or noodles to make sushi. It can also be ground up and sprinkled on grain.

Sea vegetables are also rich sources of calcium, iron, beta carotene, vitamins E, K, and the B vitamins (thiamine, riboflavin, and niacin). They even contain B12. Many are good sources of vitamin C. Nori, for example, contains 14 mg. of C; wakame, a leafy seaweed often used in soups and stews, contains 15 mg. of C. Sea vegetables also have substantial amounts of fiber and are low in fat.

If you're wondering if sea vegetables contain pollutants, have no fear. Sea vegetables are regularly tested for pollutants and consistently found to be free of all toxins. Maine Coast Sea Vegetables, one of many sea vegetable harvesters who conduct regular tests on the seaweeds they harvest, have found no traces of PCBs, hydrocarbons, and pesticides their sea vegetables. Independent authorities, such as the Maine Department of Natural Resources, confirm that the sea vegetables are safe.

"Nobody has shown that seaweeds accumulate anything toxic to any appreciable level," Dr. Mark Littler, botanist at the Smithsonian's Museum of Natural History in Washington told *The New York Times.*

Another point of concern among people is the sodium content of sea vegetables. By weight, sea vegetables do contain significant amounts of sodium, but nutritionists point out that the sodium can be reduced by rinsing and soaking the seaweeds before cooking. Also, seaweeds contain substantial amounts of potassium, the balancing electrolyte that helps to maintain the body's fluid balance. *The New York Times* reported that the sodium potassium balance in sea weeds is three parts sodium to one part potassium, very similar to the body's ratio of five parts sodium to one part potassium. Table salt, the greatest source of sodium for most people, has a ratio 10,000 parts sodium to 1 part potassium—clearly the greater threat to human health. Finally, nutritionists point out that even those who eat lots of sea vegetables do not consume them in large quantities at any one meal. Rather, they are eaten in small amounts, which provide an abundance of nutrition, but limited amounts of sodium.

Researchers at McGill University in Montreal, Canada, have found that sodium alginate, found in many seaweeds, protects bones from absorbing radioactive particles and heavy metals. Indeed, sea vegetables—long seen by scientists as an important source of nutrition in the world's future—are among the most important foods we can eat today.

AVOID THE POISONS AT ALL COSTS ○ Organic agriculture, as you know, uses no synthetic pesticides, herbicides, or fertilizers at any time during the growing, harvesting, packaging, and shipping of the foods. Only natural substances, derived directly from the earth, can be used at any stage in the growing and harvesting of organic foods. In the case of animals, organic farmers use no growth hormones and antibiotics. Only organic feed is used, and the animals are allowed to roam and live under humane conditions.

Conventional agriculture methods, on the other hand, might as well be known as petrochemical agriculture, because most of the pesticides, fertilizers, and herbicides are derived from petroleum products.

Pesticides and other environment pollutants can cause many of the common cancers, including breast cancer. The Centers for Disease Control has found that Americans now carry 100 different synthetic chemicals in their fat cells and tissues. As many as 45 of them are proven carcinogens. Many of these substances, such as atrazine and dioxin, have been shown to have an estrogen-like effect on cells, directly promoting the growth of tumors in the breast. Scientists have also discovered that low levels of these chemicals can act synergistically with each other, or be stimulated by radiation from the environment, to become even more powerful carcinogens. Researchers at the University of California at Berkeley found that dioxin levels have accumulated in human tissue over the years and, at a certain threshold, they more than double the risk of breast cancer.

Conventional livestock today are raised under the most toxic and inhumane conditions. Conventional feed contains the blood and organs of dead animals, as well as environmental pollutants, such as DDT and PCBs. The animals themselves are injected with hormones and antibiotics. And trace amounts of those same chemicals turn up in the meat and milk of these animals, and thus are consumed by humans. The animals are raised under such unhealthy conditions that they are given antibiotics to ward off disease. Unfortunately, many of the animals still suffer from such illnesses as salmonella, *E.coli*, and *listeria*. These illnesses can be passed on to humans by eating the animal's flesh and drinking its milk. Farm-raised salmon and other fish have been shown to contain high levels of growth hormones, antibiotics, and chemical pollutants, such as dioxins.

Cancer is widespread in American livestock today. Nine out of ten cows suffer from bovine leukemia virus, which not only turns up in their flesh, but also in their milk. Researchers at the University of California at Berkeley tested a community in California and found that 74 percent of those tested had been infected with the leukemia virus, according to a study published *AIDS Research and Human Retroviruses* (December 2003).

Have you ever stopped to think about how many animals contribute their flesh to a single hamburger, frankfurter, sausage, or other processed meat? Many people assume that each hamburger comes from a single cow. That's far from the truth, however. Once the cows are slaughtered, their flesh is poured into huge vats, where it is mixed together. A single vat can contain the flesh from a thousand head of cattle, which means that a single hamburger can contain the flesh from a thousand animals. The same thing happens with milk, yogurt, and cheese. It's all mixed together, causing the hormones, antibiotics, and diseases from all those animals to be homogenized into the same big container of milk and milk products.

Today's animal foods are unlike any we have eaten in human history. For those who suffer from a serious illness, the best advice is simply to avoid them.

EXERCISE IS AN ESSENTIAL PART OF A HEALING LIFESTYLE ◦ Exercise is essential to a healing way of life. It lowers weight, lowers estrogen levels, lowers insulin, increases insulin sensitivity, boosts immune function, strengthens the cancer-fighting systems, and reduces inflammation. You cannot buy any medication that can do all of that for you.

Some studies show that an hour of vigorous exercise may increase your lifespan by two years. One of the best forms of exercise is also the simplest—a daily walk. You don't have to power walk. On the contrary, just stroll if that's all you have the strength for. Take a 20 minute stroll every day. As you walk, be present and aware of your body's reaction. See if you gain energy as you walk, or become tired. If you're tired, rest for a bit, and then start again. Choose a safe distance, say, the corner of your block. Walk to that point, rest, and then walk back. Do this routine every day and watch your fitness and strength get better.

Other forms of healing exercises include yoga, gentle stretching, dancing, bicycle riding, and *Qi Gong*, a Chinese form of martial arts that scientific studies have shown to boost your immune system and fight cancer. Chinese scientists have shown that *Qi Gong* alone has been sufficient to help people overcome cancer.

A healing diet, coupled with daily exercise, can restore your health, as it did mine.

As you may know, breast cancer rates are climbing dramatically. In 1960, a woman's chance of contracting breast cancer was 1 in 20. A decade later, the risk rose to 1 in 14. Today, the American Cancer Society reports that a woman faces a 1 in 8 risk that she will contract breast cancer in her lifetime.

You can protect yourself from major illness by eating a diet that is made up primarily of whole grains, vegetables, beans, and fruit. For those who are already ill, such a diet can save your life. I am living proof of that.

○ ○ ○

COOKBOOK

RECIPES ∘ These are recipes that I used during the first two years of my macrobiotic practice. As time went on and my condition improved, I added more oil to my diet. However, these remain my core recipes.

Following the recipes is a sample month of menu plans. Also, included are some macrobiotic remedies that I used under the supervision of a macrobiotic counselor. I have listed the recipes in the following order:

Soups

Grains

Beans and bean products

Fish

Vegetables

Sea vegetables

Simple desserts

*Party foods (which I occasionally allowed myself in
    moderation on holidays, birthdays, and potlucks)*

I gradually incorporated these recipes into my family's diet. In the beginning I emptied my cupboards of most of the American processed and junk foods such as crackers, sugary baked goods, soft drinks, and candy. My children transitioned more slowly than I did. As we eliminated the sugary and artificially flavored foods from their diets, they started to eat many more vegetables, whole grains, bean products, and beans. I provided them with macrobiotic foods, but unlike me, they were free to choose from a wider assortment of foods such as occasional organic meat, eggs, cheese, and more frequent fruit-sweetened desserts. My children were provided with healthy meals at home, but had the freedom of choice outside the home—occasional school lunches or meals at a friend's or relative's house. Gradually, they learned how to make good choices. Now given the choice, they choose beans and tofu over meat and chicken, eat a variety of vegetables, and choose an apple or fruit as a snack or dessert. Over the years, they have come to embrace macrobiotic eating and as young adults can appreciate the benefits of a healthy mind and body.

SOUPS

∘ ∘ ∘

BASIC MISO SOUP
½- to 1-inch piece wakame sea vegetable per cup of soup

2 cups spring water

½-1 cup finely sliced vegetable, such as daikon radish, onion, broccoli, cauliflower, cabbage, leek, shiitake mushroom, etc. *You can any combination.*

½-1 flat teaspoon miso paste per cup of soup

2 teaspoons finely chopped scallion garnish per cup of soup

Rinse off piece of wakame and place in a small dish of water to soak until tender. Finely slice the wakame and place in a saucepan with fresh spring water. Bring to a boil (uncovered) over a medium flame.

When broth is boiling, add finely sliced vegetables, all except leafy greens. Simmer all until tender, about 3-5 minutes.

Dilute miso paste in a small amount of water, puree until smooth. Pour diluted, pureed miso into simmering broth. Add finely sliced leafy greens at this point. Simmer, *do not boil*, miso in soup for 3-4 minutes. Serve soup and garnish with chopped scallion.

CREAM OF BROCCOLI SOUP
5 cups water or stock

1 ½ cups chopped broccoli

1 small onion, diced

1½ cups cooked brown rice, or leftover oatmeal, barley or white miso

Bring water or stock to a boil. Add diced broccoli stems and onions, cover and simmer 10 minutes. Put 2 cups of the soup liquid in the blender with rice or oatmeal. Blend until smooth, then return to the pot. Add broccoli tops and simmer until tender. Flavor with miso to taste.

SQUASH AND CARROT GINGER SOUP

1 medium winter squash

6 large carrots

1 medium onion

1-inch piece ginger

4 cups water to cover veggies

sea salt, or tamari, to taste

oil if desired

Sauté onion in oil or water for 1-2 minutes. Cut up squash and carrots and add just enough water to cover the vegetables. Bring to a boil. Add a small pinch of sea salt. Cover, lower the flame and simmer 30 minutes until squash is soft.

Mash the squash with a potato masher right in the pot or use a food processor to puree. Add another pinch sea salt (or teaspoon soy sauce) and simmer 7-10 more minutes. Serve hot, garnished with fresh parsley and a little juice from grated ginger.

SPLIT PEA MISO SOUP

1 cup split peas

1 strip wakame or kombu

1 onion, diced

1 clove garlic *(optional)*

⅛ cup burdock, slivered

1 carrot or parsnip

1 stalk celery, diced

½ teaspoon thyme and marjoram

2 tablespoons barley or hatcho miso *(or more, to taste)*

Wash the peas several times, until the water is clear (makes soup less gas-forming). Boil and skim off any foam. Add seaweed, burdock, onion, and enough water to cover by 1 inch. Cover and simmer 30 minutes. Add other veggies and just enough water to make desired creaminess, simmer 30 minutes. Dissolve miso into soup just before serving.

PARSNIP SOUP

5 cups water

4 cups parsnips, cut in chunks

1 cup diced broccoli

a pinch of sea salt, or mellow miso to taste

Boil water and simmer parsnips 15 minutes or until tender. Blend until smooth, and return to the pot and add broccoli. (Thin with extra water, after blending, for desired consistency) Simmer 15-20 minutes, until broccoli is soft and the flavors have blended in to a mellow union. Season with salt, or miso, to taste.

CORN CHOWDAH

6 ears of corn

1 strip kombu

6-8 cups water

1 teaspoon corn oil

1 leek

2 carrots

½ cup corn meal

1-2 tablespoons white miso

fresh dill or parsley

Slice corn off cob. Make stock by placing cobs and kombu in pot, add water and simmer 15 minutes. Add oil, onion and leek in a large soup pot, and sauté 3 minutes over medium heat, or until onion is translucent.

Add carrots, sauté 3 minutes. Add corn, sauté 1 minute.

Sprinkle corn meal and stir well so veggies are coated. When mixture begins to turn golden, strain cobs from stock and add stock to soup pot stirring quickly to prevent lumps.

Place on flame tamer and simmer ½ hour. Dissolve miso and simmer 3-4 minutes or add sea salt and cook 12 minutes. Garnish with dill or basil.

BLACK BEAN SOUP

1 cup black beans, soaked overnight and covered with water

4 cups water

6-inch strip kombu seaweed

2 cups chopped cauliflower

1 carrot, diced

1 teaspoon finely grated ginger

pinch cumin *(optional)*

1 green onion, sliced

2-3 teaspoons tamari soy sauce

Wash and soak black beans overnight. Drain soaking water and add fresh. Place in the pressure cooker with kombu, bring to pressure, and simmer for 1 hour (or pot boil for 1½ hours).

Bring down from pressure. Add cauliflower, ginger, carrot and cumin and simmer 20 minutes—just until veggies are tender. Stir in the green onion, season with tamari, and let it sit awhile before serving, to let the flavors blend.

Garnish with slivers of fresh green onion. Tastes even better the next day.

Variation. If available, include 2 collard leaves, sliced (add with cauliflower)

MUSHROOM BARLEY SOUP

1 cup whole barley, soaked overnight and covered with water

1 teaspoon light sesame oil

1 onion, sliced thin half moons

5-6 cups mushroom stock

4-5 dried shiitake mushrooms, soaked until tender, thinly sliced

1 cup button mushrooms, brushed free of dirt, thinly sliced

soy sauce

2 ribs celery, thinly sliced

fresh scallions, thinly sliced for garnish

Rinse the barley by placing it in a bowl and covering with water. Swirl gently and drain. After soaking the barley, drain and discard the soaking water.

In a soup pot, heat oil and sauté onions until translucent. Add stock and barley and bring to a boil over high heat. Stir in mushrooms. Reduce heat and cook, covered, for about 40 minutes until barley becomes soft and creamy.

Season lightly with soy sauce and simmer for 10-15 minutes more.

Stir in raw celery for some crunch and serve garnished with fresh scallions.

Note. You may use pearled barley, a cracked form of the whole grain.

ADZUKI BEAN VEGETABLE SOUP

1-inch piece kombu

1 cup adzuki beans, sorted, rinsed and soaked overnight and covered with water

7-8 cups spring or filtered water

1 sweet onion, diced

1 cup green head cabbage, diced

1 cup winter squash, diced

1-2 stalks celery, diced

1 cup fresh/frozen corn kernels

3-4 teaspoons barley miso (¼–½ teaspoon per cup of liquid)

2-3 fresh scallions, thinly sliced on the diagonal, for garnish

Place kombu on the bottom of a heavy soup pot. Top with beans, discarding soaking water. Add water and bring to a boil, uncovered.

Allow beans to cook for 5 minutes over high heat. Cover, reduce heat to low and simmer until beans are about 85% done, 35-40 minutes.

Add vegetables, return soup to a boil, reduce heat to low and simmer until both beans and vegetables are soft, 40 minutes. Add miso, cook 3-4 minutes. Garnish with scallions.

MILLET-SWEET VEGETABLE SOUP

½ cup millet, rinsed well

¼ cup each onion, carrot, winter squash, green cabbage, finely diced

5 cups spring or filtered water

2 teaspoons barley miso

1-2 fresh scallions, thinly sliced for garnish

Rinse millet by placing in a glass bowl and covering with water. Gently swirl grain with your hands to loosen any dust. Drain well.

In a soup pot, layer onion, cabbage, squash, carrot and then millet. Add enough water to just cover, careful not to disturb layering too much. Cover and bring to a boil over medium heat.

Reduce heat, simmer for 30 minutes. Remove a small amount of broth and puree the miso. Gently stir into the soup and simmer for another 3-4 minutes. Garnish with fresh scallions.

BROCCOLI-NOODLE SOUP

1 teaspoon light or dark sesame oil

1 medium onion, cut into thin crescents

1 medium bunch broccoli, cut stem in quarter rounds and flowerets into 2-inch pieces

8 cups boiling water

¼ teaspoon sea salt

2 cups whole wheat ribbon noodles, lightly packed

1 or 2 tablespoons of sesame butter (optional, but yummy)

2-3 tablespoons soy sauce

Heat oil in large, heavy saucepan over medium heat. Add onions and sauté until transparent, 1-2 minutes. Add broccoli stems and sauté 1 minute. Add boiling water and sea salt, cover, bring to a boil, lower heat and simmer 10 minutes. Add noodles and broccoli flowerets.

Cover and simmer 15 minutes. Dilute sesame butter in ¼ cup hot soup broth, add to soup with soy sauce, stir to heat through but do not boil.

MINESTRONE SOUP

¾ cup cannelini beans

¾ cup kidney beans

¾ cup lentils

onion

3 carrots, diced

½ lb. green beans

celery, 3 stalks, diced

corn, 1 package

parsley (1 cup)

¼ - ½ cup ume plum vinegar

2 cups of cooked whole wheat pasta

Soak cannelini beans and kidney beans overnight. Prepare vegetables.

Cook beans in a pressure cooker according to your instructions or cook on stovetop by covering with water and bringing to a boil, turning to low and cooking for 1 ½ - 2 hours or until soft. Just before beans are done, add vegetables, bring to a boil again, and cook 10 -15 minutes (you may need to add extra water).

When beans and vegetables are done, add 1 tablespoon ume plum vinegar (depending on size of soup) and whole wheat pasta.

NOODLES IN BROTH

½ pack udon or soba noodles

1 shiitake mushroom

1-inch piece kombu

½ onion, sliced in half moons

1-inch piece burdock, cut in matchsticks

1-inch piece carrot, cut in matchsticks

1-inch summer squash, sliced thinly on a diagonal

1 stalk celery, sliced finely on a diagonal

2-4 ounces tofu, cubed

2-3 tablespoons shoyu

mirin *(optional)*

brown rice vinegar *(optional)*

2 teaspoons kuzu *(optional)*

grated ginger

1 tablespoon roasted sesame seeds

nori, cut very fine

bonito flakes *(optional)*

scallions, sliced for garnish

10 cups of water

Cook noodles in separate pot. Rinse and set aside. Put kombu and shiitake in water and bring to a boil. Simmer 10-20 minutes.

Remove kombu and shiitake, slice both into strips and return to broth. Add onion, burdock and carrots, let simmer 10 minutes.

Add summer squash, celery, tofu and shoyu to taste—approximately 1 teaspoon per cup of liquid. Add other seasonings—½ as much mirin as shoyu and just a dash of brown rice vinegar. Let it all simmer 5 more minutes.

Dilute kuzu in cold water. Add to broth, stirring constantly to avoid lumping. Bring to a boil, then back to simmer. Pour over pre-cooked noodles. Serve with ginger, scallions, sesame seeds, bonito flakes and nori as garnishes.

HOT AND SOUR SOUP

¼ pound seitan, shredded

½ teaspoon soy sauce, plus additional to taste

1 teaspoon mirin

2 teaspoons kuzu

2 teaspoon sesame oil

1-2 teaspoons hot pepper sesame oil *(optional)*

1 small onion, cut into very thin half-moon slices

4 dried shiitake mushrooms, soaked until tender, thinly sliced

3-4 button mushrooms, thinly sliced

4-5 cups spring or filtered water

1 broccoli stalk, peeled and cut into fine matchstick pieces

½ pound extra-firm tofu, cut into tiny cubes

1 tablespoon kuzu dissolved in 2 tablespoons cold water

1-2 tablespoons umeboshi vinegar

2-3 scallions, thinly sliced, for garnish

Cut seitan into matchsticks and place in a medium bowl. Combine ½ teaspoon soy sauce, mirin, kuzu and sesame oil in a small bowl. Toss with the seitan pieces, set aside.

Over medium flame, heat hot pepper sesame oil in a soup pot. Add onion, sauté until translucent, about 2 minutes. Add mushrooms and sauté 1-2 minutes. Stir in seitan, sauté briefly. Add water, cover, and bring to a boil over medium heat.

Stir in broccoli and tofu cubes. Cover and simmer 20-25 minutes. Season to taste with soy sauce, simmer for 5-7 minutes. Stir in dissolved kuzu until soup thickens slightly about 3 minutes.

Remove soup from heat and season lightly with vinegar to taste. Serve hot, garnished with scallions.

GRAINS

○ ○ ○

BOILED RICE
2 cups organic short grain brown rice

4 cups spring water

small pinch sea salt

Soak 1-2 cups organic brown rice for 3-5 hours, or overnight, in spring water. Use 2 parts water per 1 part rice. Place rice and its soaking water in a pot, bring to a boil over medium flame. When gently boiling, add a pinch of sea salt or 1-inch square piece dry kombu. Cover the pot with a heavy lid, lower the flame, simmer for 45-50 minutes. When finished, allow the rice to sit for 3-5 minutes undisturbed before removing the cover. Uncover and place rice in a separate serving bowl, cover with a cotton cloth or bamboo mat until ready to eat.

Variation. Cook rice with either 30% barley, millet, rye, oats, corn off the cob or wheat berries.

BROWN RICE WITH BARLEY-PRESSURE COOKED
2 cups organic brown rice, washed and soaked overnight and covered with water

1 cup whole barley, washed and soaked overnight and covered with water

4½ cups water, including soaking water from barley

small pinch sea salt, or piece kombu soaked and diced

Place brown rice, barley and water in pressure cooker. Place over low flame and bring to boil, add salt, cover, turn up flame to high and bring to pressure. Reduce flame to medium low, place on flame deflector and cook 45-50 minutes.

Remove from flame and allow pressure to come down naturally. Place in serving bowl and serve.

PRESSURE COOKED RICE AND BEANS

1½ to 1¾ cups brown rice

½ cup beans (chickpeas, adzuki, black soybean, etc.) soaked overnight and covered with water

3½ to 4 cups spring water

small piece kombu sea vegetable

Use 10-15% beans per cup of rice, pre-soak either adzuki, chickpeas, black soybeans or other bean of your choice for 3-7 hours depending on the hardness of the bean. Discard the soak water, for any but adzuki or black soybeans, and mix beans with rice.

Place rice and bean mixture in pressure cooker, add water (1½ to 2 parts water for every 1 cup of grain and bean you have combined) and bring to a gentle boil.

When boiling add a 1- to 2-inch piece kombu, seal the lid and bring to pressure over a medium flame. When the full pressure rises in the pot, lower the flame, place on a flame deflector and cook for 45-50 minutes. When finished, turn off flame and remove from heat.

Allow the pressure to come down naturally and remove the lid. Transfer to a serving bowl.

Note. Include the soaking water from black soy or adzuki beans. Do not add salt to this recipe at the beginning or the skin of the beans will not soften.

MILLET WITH SWEET VEGETABLES
1 cup millet
1 cup hard winter squash or equal volume of sweet vegetables
3 cups spring water
pinch sea salt

Place millet, squash and spring water in a pot. Bring to a boil over medium flame, add sea salt and cover.

Lower flame, place on a flame deflector, simmer 35 minutes. Remove millet from heat and place in a serving bowl.

Note. Corn, onions, peas, cabbage, carrots, parsnips, leeks, turnips and rutabagas also work well in this dish.

MORNING PORRIDGE FROM LEFTOVER GRAIN
1 cup leftover cooked whole grain
2-3 cups fresh spring water

Place grain and water in a pot. Bring to a boil. Cover and simmer over a low flame for 15 minutes or until grain reaches porridge-like consistency.

Serve garnished with chopped parsley, a pinch of condiment, a piece of umeboshi plum, etc.

Note. Occasionally sweeten morning porridge with a spoonful of rice syrup, barley malt, or some amasake. Cook in some fruit like raisins or apples into the porridge occasionally.

WHOLE OATS PORRIDGE

Soak whole oaks in the morning, cook them in the evening and reheat (in a little water) the next morning for cereal.

1 cup whole oats groats* soaked overnight in 6-7 cups water
pinch sea salt or small piece kombu or ¼ cup dulse

Place the oats and soaking water in a pot and add the salt or sea vegetable. Cover and bring to a boil over a medium flame. Reduce flame to low and simmer for 1-1½ hours, or longer, until oats are tender and creamy. Serve garnished with condiment, raisins or toasted seeds.

Whole oatmeal that we buy is run through a roller, so it is a "cracked" grain. Whole oat groats are even heartier than regular oatmeal and look like rice until they are cooked—then they soften and open. I soak them overnight and then cook them. They are especially good for eating during the winter.

PAN FRIED MOCHI

½-1 package brown rice or mugwort mochi
2-3 tablespoons fresh grated daikon
1 scallion, sliced
soy sauce

Slice mochi into 1- to 2-inch squares. Heat a cast iron or heavy skillet over a medium flame.

When the pan is hot, reduce flame to absolutely lowest point and place mochi in the pan. Cover, cook over low flame for 4 minutes.

Lift cover, gently turn mochi over, replace cover and cook 2-4 minutes longer. When mochi puffs slightly, remove from pan and serve with a garnish of grated daikon radish mixed with several drops of shoyu and some chopped scallion.

MOCHI WAFFLES WITH MIXED BERRY SAUCE
1 (8-ounce) package brown rice mochi

Heat a nonstick, Belgian waffle iron. While the iron warms, slice the mochi into ⅛-inch-thick strips. When the iron is hot, lay the strips, loosely touching, in the waffle iron. You will need to press firmly to close the iron. Cook waffles 1 minute for softer waffles, up to 2 minutes for crispier ones.

Mixed Berry Sauce

2 cups unfiltered apple juice or spring or filtered water

pinch of sea salt

¼ cup fresh strawberries, quartered

¼ cup fresh blueberries

¼ cup fresh raspberries

¼ cup fresh cherries, pitted and halved

1 tablespoon kuzu, dissolved in 4 tablespoons cold water

dash of pure vanilla extract

Bring juice and salt to a boil in a saucepan over medium heat. Stir in fruit and simmer over low heat 5-7 minutes, until fruit softens. Stir in dissolved kuzu and cook, stirring until mixture thickens slightly, about 3 minutes.

QUINOA
1 cup quinoa

2¼ cups water

pinch sea salt

Wash quinoa or rinse well through strainer. Roast in skillet, stirring until nutty smelling. Add water, bring to a boil, cover and simmer 20 minutes.

Variation. Add diced onion or 3 tablespoons sesame or sunflower seeds.

GRAIN SALAD

1 cup leftover, cooked whole or cracked grain such as barley or bulgur wheat

¼ cup red radishes sliced finely

¼ cup finely sliced or diced cucumber

1 scallion or handful chives finely sliced

¼ cup finely diced carrot, blanched quickly in boiling water

1 ear corn-on-the-cob, kernels shaved and blanched quickly in boiling water

2 tablespoons umeboshi vinegar or other dressing

Toss all ingredients together and enjoy at room temperature or chilled for a light grain entrée.

GENUINE BROWN RICE CREAM

1 cup organic short grain brown rice

10 cups fresh spring water

pinch sea salt

Dry roast rice in a cast iron, or stainless steel, skillet until golden. Place the rice in a pot and add 10 cups of spring water. Add pinch of sea salt. Bring to a boil on a medium to high flame.

Cover, lower the flame and slide a flame deflector under pot. Cook for 1½-2 hours until the water has reduced by half. Remove pot from flame, remove soft rice and allow to cool.

Place the soft rice in a cheesecloth or fine mesh strainer and squeeze out the cream. Serve garnished with a small amount of condiment such as gomasio or piece of umeboshi plum.

Note. Use genuine brown rice cream as a breakfast cereal or for any sickness where it is difficult to chew, swallow or keep food down.

MISO-VEGETABLE SOFT GRAIN PORRIDGE
1 cup leftover rice or other grain

2-3 cups spring water

½ small onion, diced

1 tablespoon scallion roots, diced

½ cup cauliflower, cut in small pieces

2 teaspoons 2-year aged miso, diluted in ¼ cup water

1 sheet toasted nori for garnish

2 teaspoons sliced fresh scallions for garnish

Place the vegetables, rice, and water in a saucepan and bring to a boil over a medium flame. Reduce flame to low and simmer 15-20 minutes.

When mixture is creamy and vegetables tender add the diluted miso and simmer 4 minutes. Serve hot, garnished with nori and scallions.

Variation: Simmer grain alone first, then sauté vegetables in oil and add to the soft grain along with miso for a richer stew.

JESSICA'S "HAMBURGER" HELPER
1 cup whole grain elbows

1 cup bulgur

1 package tempeh

veggies – mushrooms, corn, onions, broccoli

shoyu to taste (1 teaspoon)

sesame oil for frying (1 teaspoon)

3 cups water

Sauté veggies in oil. Add dry pasta and bulgur, sauté several minutes. Cover with water, add tempeh, bring to a boil, and let simmer 20 minutes. Add shoyu.

CORN POLENTA (BASIC PREPARATION)
1 cup coarse ground corn meal

4 cups water

¼ cup water

¼ teaspoon sea salt

Bring 4 cups of water to a boil. Very slowly whisk in 1 cup of polenta, simmer and stir frequently for 5-10 minutes until very thick. Tasted delicious served warm.

Variation. Place in bread pan and chill for 2 hours. Slice and prepare as desired.

GOMASIO
8 round tablespoons organic unhulled (tan or black) sesame seeds

1½ teaspoons unrefined white sea salt

Wash seeds in a fine mesh strainer and allow to drain. Dry roast the sea salt in a stainless steel skillet over a medium flame until it is shiny. Transfer salt to a suribachi and grind into a fine powder.

Roast the seeds on a medium flame stirring constantly with a wooden spatula. When the seeds begin to pop, darken, give off a nutty aroma and crush easily between thumb and forefinger they are done.

Promptly add the seeds to the suribachi on top of the ground, roasted salt and grind in a steady circular motion until 85-90% crushed into a fluffy powder, thoroughly coating the salt. Store in a tightly sealed glass jar.

Note. The standard ratio of sesame seeds to sea salt is 16 or 18 to 1. Prepare this condiment fresh at home every 7-10 days. Store it in a sealed glass jar. Use black or tan seeds.

RICE BALLS
1 sheet toasted nori
2 cups cooked rice
1 umeboshi plum torn in two pieces

Fold the full sheet of nori in half, tear cleanly into two pieces. Fold each piece in half and tear into 2 pieces—resulting in 4, 3-inch squares.

Moisten your palms with either lightly salted water or bancha tea. Place about ¾ cup rice in one hand.

Form the rice into a flat triangle by cupping your hands into a "v" and applying pressure to mold the rice. The triangle should be firmly packed.

With one finger press a hole into the center of the rice and insert half an umeboshi plum. Close the hole by packing the triangle firmly again.

Place one square of nori on one side of the triangle and pack it well, until it sticks. Repeat with another square of nori on the uncovered side of the triangle.

Make sure every inch of rice is covered with nori, especially if you intend to take these on a trip and carry them unrefrigerated for any period of time. Well-made rice balls will last for up to 3 days.

Variations. Instead of covering the balls in nori, roll them in toasted seeds or roasted, chopped nuts, or whole shiso leaves.
Use other grains to make the balls.
Pan fry the rice balls in a little oil for a rich taste.
Use takuan or other pickle in the center, sometimes umeboshi.

BEANS

○ ○ ○

TEMPEH TUNA

1 package (8 ounces) tempeh

1 stalk celery, diced fine

½ red onion, diced fine

1 cup Nayonnaise or tofu mayo *(see next page)*

2 teaspoons brown rice syrup

2 tablespoons, then ½ teaspoon, umeboshi vinegar

2 teaspoons brown rice vinegar

½ teaspoon lemon juice

cumin, turmeric or curry *(optional)*

Steam or boil tempeh 20 minutes. Mash it with a fork or potato masher.

Dilute 2 tablespoons umeboshi vinegar in ½ cup of water and pour over tempeh. Mix into tempeh with your hands, so that the tempeh becomes saturated in the mixture.

In a bowl, mix nayonnaise, umeboshi vinegar, brown rice vinegar, lemon juice and brown rice syrup. Whisk together and taste.

If you prefer any one taste over another, increase that ingredient. Add pepper to taste. *(Options: cumin, turmeric, curry)*

TOFU MAYONNAISE

8 ounce tofu

½ cup water

2 teaspoons sesame or olive oil

1 tablespoon lemon juice

1 tablespoon brown rice vinegar

1 tablespoon mellow white miso (or ¼ teaspoon sea salt)

sprinkle of dill *(optional)*

Slice tofu; steam 3 minutes. Blend ingredients until smooth and creamy.

Note. This keeps refrigerated for 2-3 days, If it separates, just re-blend.

SWEET AND SOUR PINTO BEANS

1 cup pinto beans, soaked overnight and covered with water

3 cups water

1-inch piece kombu

1 large onion, diced

1 carrot, diced

shoyu

2 tablespoons barley malt

1-2 teaspoons stone-ground mustard

umeboshi vinegar

Drain beans, then pressure cook with kombu 50 minutes. Allow pressure to come down, then add vegetables, and cook 20 minutes.

Add several shakes of shoyu and barley malt, cook 10 minutes. Add umeboshi vinegar and mustard.

BLACK SOYBEAN STEW

1 cup black soybeans, soaked overnight and covered with water

1 onion, diced

1 carrot, diced

½ cup fresh or dried lotus root, sliced

½ cup minced burdock or squash, finely diced for burdock, cubed for squash

1 stalk celery, diced

½ cup dried daikon soaked for 10 minutes, save and use soaking water

3-5 pieces dried tofu soaked, rinsed and sliced

2-inch strip kombu, rinsed

½ teaspoon sea salt

1 tablespoon soy sauce

1 tablespoon barley malt

Place the kombu on the bottom of a pressure cooker and add the black soybeans together with their soaking water.

Bring beans to a boil over a medium flame. Leave the pot uncovered.

Reduce the flame to low and simmer uncovered for 30 minutes, adding fresh spring water as needed to keep the water levels with the beans.

After approximately 30 minutes, add ¼ cup water, cover the pressure cooker, raise the flame and bring to pressure on a medium-high flame.

Reduce flame, place a flame deflector under the pot and pressure cook 45 minutes. Bring pressure down in the pot by pouring cold water over pot or by placing cold towels on the lid.

Open pot, pour out beans into a bowl and layer in the vegetables in the following order: celery, onion, squash, carrot, lotus root, burdock, dried daikon.

Pour the beans on top of the vegetables, then layer the dried tofu on top.

Bring the pot to a boil over a medium flame. Cover, reduce flame, cook 30 minutes.

Add the sea salt and cook another 5-7 minutes. Add soy sauce and barley malt and cook another 5-7 minutes.

Gently mix stew by swirling the pot. Remove from flame and serve in a large bowl garnished with minced parsley.

BAKED BEANS WITH MISO AND APPLE BUTTER

2 cups kidney beans, soaked overnight and covered with water

6 cups water

1 strip kombu

1½ tablespoons mellow barley miso

¼ cup unsweetened apple butter

1½ teaspoons whole grain mustard

1 tablespoon grated onion

⅔ tablespoon brown rice vinegar

Cook beans with kombu in water for 45 minutes. Drain and save 1 cup of the cooking water. Preheat oven to 350°.

Oil a 3-quart casserole. Mix everything, except the beans, with the cooking liquid and then mix in beans. Cover and bake for 1½ hour.

NATTO (FERMENTED SOYBEANS) CONDIMENT

½ cup organic natto

3 tablespoons finely sliced, fresh scallion

1 sheet toasted nori, torn into small pieces

½ teaspoon yellow mustard *(optional)*

1 tablespoon soy sauce, or to taste

Using a fork, whip the natto in a bowl until frothy. Mix in scallions, nori and soy sauce. Whip together well. If adding mustard, add here and mix in well. Serve a couple of spoonfuls on top of rice or noodles.

Note. Unseasoned natto may also be chopped on a cutting board and added to miso soup at a ratio of about 1-2 teaspoons per bowl. Natto is usually found in the refrigerator section of the natural foods or Oriental grocery. Keep it chilled or frozen until ready to serve. It will store refrigerated for up to one month.

GINGERED CHICKPEAS
2 cups of chickpeas
1 onion
sea salt
parsley
fresh ginger
potato masher

Cover 2 cups of chickpeas with water and soak overnight. Drain soaking water. Put chickpeas in a pot and add water to cover an inch or more.

Peel onion and place in middle of chickpeas. Bring to a boil, cover, turn to low, and simmer for 1 - 1 ¼ hours.

Add ¼ teaspoon sea salt, and simmer 10 more minutes.

When done, pour off a cup or so of the cooking water and set aside. This can be used to thin soup if too thick.

Take the potato masher and mash chickpeas and onion until ½ of the peas are pureed.

Grate some ginger and squeeze the juice into the mixture to taste. Garnish with freshly chopped parsley.

Serve plain or on top of brown rice.

CHICKPEA BURGERS

1½ cup chickpeas, soaked overnight and covered with water

4½ cups water

1-inch piece kombu

½ cup rolled oats

2 organic dill pickles, diced

1 small carrot, diced

1 red onion, minced

1 tablespoon rice syrup

1 teaspoon mustard

1 teaspoon white miso

1 teaspoon umeboshi vinegar

corn meal for coating

Pressure cook chickpeas with kombu in water for 40 minutes. Mash cooked chickpeas, add balance of ingredients, shape into patties and coat with corn meal.

Let the patties sit for 20 minutes, then fry in a cast iron skillet on medium heat until browned on each side. Serve plain, or with a sauce, on steamed bread.

SQUASH ADZUKI BEANS AND CHESTNUTS

1 cup adzuki beans, soaked overnight and covered with water

1 strip kombu

1 small butternut or buttercup squash

1 cup soaked chestnuts (*optional*)

tamari or sea salt to taste (⅛ teaspoon of salt)

Place kombu on the bottom of a medium pot (with lid). Add squash, cut in ½- to 1-inch cubes, chestnuts, with their soaking water, and beans, without soaking water.

Cover with water. Bring to a boil, simmer 1 hour. Add sea salt or tamari to taste. Cook uncovered 15 minutes or until liquid boils off.

TEMPEH WITH SAUERKRAUT AND ONIONS

½-1 cup tempeh, cut into 2-inch cubes

2 onions, sliced into thin half moons

½ cup cabbage, finely sliced

1 cup spring water

½ cup sauerkraut

2 tablespoons sauerkraut juice

1 teaspoon soy sauce

1 tablespoon mirin (*optional*)

1 tablespoon minced, fresh parsley

Heat a skillet over medium high flame. Add a few drops water and lightly sauté onions until shiny and soft. Add cabbage and sauté 2 minutes.

Add tempeh and add water to almost cover. Cover pan, reduce flame to low, simmer 15 minutes.

Add sauerkraut, its juice and soy sauce, simmer 5 minutes. If using mirin, add here.

Serve immediately and garnish with chopped parsley.

SCRAMBLED (SAUTÉED) TOFU WITH VEGETABLES

1 block (pound) firm tofu, coarsely mashed with a fork or crumbled by hand

1 onion, finely diced

1 carrot, finely diced

1 ear fresh, sweet corn, kernels shaved off the cob

1 scallion, finely sliced

sesame oil

soy sauce

spring water

Heat a skillet over medium flame and brush the bottom with oil Add onions, and sauté until shiny.

Add carrots, and sauté 1-2 minutes.

Add corn, sauté 1 minute.

Add tofu, mix with the vegetables.

Add water, if necessary, to prevent sticking.

Cover skillet, reduce flame to low and steam for 1 minute.

Add 1-2 teaspoons soy sauce, mix well, cover and steam for 3 minutes.

Serve immediately and garnish with chopped scallion.

FISH

∘ ∘ ∘

FISH STEW (GOOD AFTER SKIING)
1 medium onion
1 carrot
1 stalk celery
3 cups cooked brown rice (or other whole grain)
6 cups water
1 pound white meat fish (with no bones)
1 tablespoon grated fresh ginger root
2 tablespoons shoyu or 1 teaspoon sea salt
3 tablespoons chopped parsley for garnish

Mince the onion, carrot and celery.

Place them in a 4-quart saucepan along with the rice and water.

Cover and simmer for 20 minutes, stirring often.

Rinse the fish under cold running water and pat dry. Cut each fillet into several large pieces and add to pot, along with the ginger and shoyu.

Cover the pot and simmer for 10-15 minutes.

Garnish with parsley.

STEAMED HADDOCK

1½ pounds haddock, washed and cut into 4-5 equal-sized pieces

4-5 broccoli flowerets, washed

¼ cup carrots, washed, sliced in thick matchsticks or flower shapes

spring or well water

3 lemons sliced for garnish

1 cup tamari-ginger dip sauce

Place the fish in a ceramic bowl. Attractively arrange the broccoli and carrots in the bowl with the fish.

Set the bowl down inside a large pot, with about ½ inch of water in the pot. Cover the pot and bring the water to a boil.

Steam for several minutes until the fish is tender and the vegetables are brightly colored and tender.

Remove, garnish with lemon slices, and serve with the tamari-ginger dip sauce.

Tamari-Ginger Dip Sauce

¼ teaspoon grated ginger

1 tablespoon shoyu

¼ cup of spring or well water

Mix ingredients and heat up. Serve in a small cup or bowl.

CARP BURDOCK SOUP – KOI KOKU

1, 2-pound carp

2 pounds (or equal weight to weight of fish) burdock root shaved or sliced into matchstick

¾ -1 cup used bancha or kukicha twigs

cheesecloth/cotton string

sesame oil

spring water and bancha tea

barley miso

freshly grated ginger root

chopped fresh scallions

Buy a fresh carp. Ask the fish seller to carefully remove the gallbladder and yellow bitter bone (thyroid) and leave the rest of the fish intact, with all scales, bones, head and fins.

At home, chop the entire fish into two or three inch slices. Remove the eyes if you wish. Chop an amount of burdock equal to the weight of the fish into thinly shaved slices or matchsticks.

Optional step. Sauté the burdock for a few minutes in sesame oil and place the fish on top of the burdock in a pressure cooker.

Tie cooked (used) kukicha twigs (about one cup) in a cheese cloth. Place it in the pressure cooker on top or nestled inside the fish. The tea twigs will help soften the bones.

Add enough liquid to cover the fish and burdock, approximately one-third bancha tea and two thirds spring water. Pressure cook for 1½-2 hours.

Bring the pressure down, remove the lid and replace on a low flame. Add miso to taste and a small amount of ginger juice. Simmer for 5 minutes.

Garnish with chopped scallions, serve hot.

VEGETABLES

○ ○ ○

QUICK STEAMED GREENS

1-2 cups leafy greens*, washed carefully and sliced

spring water

Wash and slice any combination of leafy greens. Bring water to a rapid boil over a high flame in a pot or steamer pan. Add greens, cover and steam on high for 2-3 minutes, depending on the texture of the leaves. Remove from pan immediately and place on a flat platter to stop them from cooking longer.

kale, collard greens, or mustard greens

BOILED SALAD — BLANCHED VEGETABLES

1 cup thinly sliced Chinese cabbage

½ cup thinly sliced leek

1 cup broccoli flowerets

¼ cup summer squash sliced into half rounds

5-6 red radishes, halved

Fill a pot half full with spring water. Bring to a rolling boil over a medium to high flame. Place each vegetable one at a time in water and boil uncovered only until the color turns bright, one minute or less.

Blanch each vegetable separately and in order from mildest to strongest tasting so that each retains its own distinct flavor and color. Use a fine mesh skimmer to remove the vegetables from the boiling water.

Drain each vegetable on a flat surface to stop cooking. Serve blanched salad plain, with dressing, or a splash of vinegar or lemon juice. Serve warm, at room temperature or chilled, tossed together or arranged in sections on a platter.

STEAMED ROOTS AND TOPS

½ large bunch carrots and their green tops*

spring water

soy sauce

Separate the roots from their green tops. Finely slice the roots and place in a pot with a small amount of water.

Cover, cook with high steam for 5 minutes, or until roots are firm but tender.

Add a few drops of soy sauce or umeboshi vinegar to the roots. Add finely sliced green tops, re-cover the pot and steam 2-3 minutes.

Remove from flame when root greens are still bright and serve promptly.

For carrots, I don't use the woody stick part between the carrot and leaves

LIGHTLY STEAMED VEGETABLES

seitan, tempeh, fresh or dried tofu

root and leafy green vegetables

Place seitan, tempeh, fresh or dried tofu, root and leafy green vegetables in sections around a pot.

Add enough water to cover the bottom of the pot. Add a few drops of soy sauce or pinch of salt. Cover and steam on a medium-high flame for 4-5 minutes.

Quick cooking leafy greens such as scallions or watercress may be added closer to the end of cooking. Serve right from the pot.

LONG, SLOW STEAMING (NISHIME STYLE)
1 carrot cut into large chunks
¼ cabbage cut into large wedges
1 onion sliced into large wedges
¼ cup hard, sweet winter squash cubed
¼ cup daikon sliced into large chunks
2-3 inch strip kombu soaked and sliced into small strips

Place kombu and its soaking water in the bottom of a pot. Layer the vegetables on top of one another in the following order: daikon, onion, cabbage, squash and carrot (burdock and lotus root may be cut smaller).

Cover pot and bring to a boil over a medium high flame until there is steam from the pot. Lower flame and cook without disturbing the pot for 15-20 minutes or longer. If water evaporates during cooking add more water to the bottom of the pot.

When vegetables have become tender, add a few drops of soy sauce and mix. Replace cover and simmer five more minutes. Remove from the flame, let sit, and serve after a couple minutes.

Vary the combinations of vegetables each time you prepare the dish.

Try these combinations:
• turnip, onion, carrot, shiitake
• carrot, leek, cauliflower, corn, daikon, shiitake, daikon greens
• burdock, carrot, onion, squash

LONG SAUTÉ AND SIMMERED ROOTS — KINPIRA

1 large carrot sliced into thin matchsticks
1 medium burdock root sliced into thin matchsticks
toasted sesame oil
soy sauce
½ teaspoon juice from freshly grated ginger

Lightly brush the skillet with sesame oil or add water and heat.

Place vegetables in the skillet and add a pinch of sea salt. Sauté for 3-4 minutes.

Add water to lightly cover bottom of the skillet. Cover and simmer vegetables for 15 minutes or longer until vegetables are tender.

Add several drops of soy sauce, cover again and cook until all the water has cooked down. At the very end of cooking, add a few drops of ginger juice.

LIGHTLY STEWED VEGETABLES WITH TOFU, DRIED TOFU, TEMPEH OR SEITAN

2 inches kombu, soaked and thinly sliced

1 carrot cut into bite sized chunks

¼ cup cauliflower

½ onion sliced into half moons

½ cup Napa cabbage

3 scallions sliced into long strips

½ cup fresh tofu cut into 1 inch cubes

spring water

soy sauce

Layer kombu, carrot and cauliflower in a pot Add enough water to cover the vegetables.

Bring to a boil over a medium flame and simmer for about 3 minutes. Season lightly with soy sauce.

Add onion, Napa, and tofu and cook for another 3-5 minutes.

Add scallions and cook for 1 more minute. All vegetables should be cooked until tender but the leafy greens should still be bright and crisp.

Serve vegetables with the broth.

SQUASH, ADZUKI BEANS, & KOMBU

1 cup adzuki beans, rinsed and soaked overnight and covered with water

2 cups sweet, winter squash cut into 2-3 inch cubes

2-3 inch piece kombu, soaked and sliced into squares

sea salt

Place kombu on bottom of heavy pot. Add the squash, then pour the beans and their soaking water over the squash.

Bring the water level equal with the squash and bring to a boil over a low flame. Cover the pot. Watch to see that the beans sink down beneath the water level. If necessary add fresh water to just cover the beans.

Cook over a low flame for about 1 hour or until the beans and squash become soft. Open the pot and season lightly with sea salt (about ⅛ teaspoon per cup of dry beans.)

Let salt cook in 10-25 minutes. If extra liquid remains leave pot uncovered and simmer off liquid.

Remove from flame and let sit several minutes before serving.

DRIED DAIKON RADISH WITH VEGETABLES & KOMBU
½ cup dried daikon, soaked until tender and sliced
(if it is very dark in color discard its soaking water)
1-2 shiitake mushrooms, soaked and sliced finely
1 onion sliced into half moons
2 inch strip kombu soaked and sliced into thin strips
spring water

Soak kombu and dried daikon separately until tender enough to slice.

Slice kombu lengthwise into thin strips and place on the bottom of a pot. Slice dried daikon into bite sized pieces. (If it is very dark in color discard its soaking water.)

Layer the shiitake on top of the daikon and the onions on top of the shiitake.

Add the dried daikon and cover all with a combination of fresh spring water and the soaking waters from the shiitake, kombu and dried daikon.

Bring to a boil over a medium flame, lower flame, cover and simmer 30-40 minutes.

Open pot, season with a small amount of soy sauce and cook away any remaining liquid.

Serve warm garnished with a small amount of fresh parsley or scallion.

NABE STYLE VEGETABLES

¼-½ cup each of at least 5-7 vegetables

(cut into bite-sized pieces and arranged in sections on a platter.

Emphasize upward growing and leafy types)

A typical combination would be:

leek

Chinese cabbage

bok choy

snow peas

brussel sprouts

summer squash

white mushrooms

bean sprouts

shiitake mushroom

1-inch piece kombu sea vegetable

spring water

Bring 2-3 cups of water, the shiitake and kombu to a boil in a wide, shallow pan or ceramic nabe pot. Place the pot on a portable burner on the dining table. Each person may select vegetables and other items from the raw platter, place them in the boiling water or kombu broth and simmer briefly until bright.

Eat these vegetables immediately with a dipping sauce and side dish of grain.

Nabe Dip

2 teaspoons soy sauce

3-4 tablespoons water or cooking broth

¼ teaspoon fresh ginger

½ teaspoon rice vinegar or lemon juice

Mix and place in a small bowl large enough for dipping vegetables. *Note.* Dipping sauces may include cooking broth with soy sauce and rice vinegar or ginger juice added. Nabe vegetables comprise ⅔ of a nabe meal, ⅓ of the meal may be a grain dish such as noodles or rice.

QUICK SAUTÉED VEGETABLES
¼ cup leek, finely sliced
¼ cup cabbage, shredded
¼ cup mushrooms, thinly sliced
¼ cup thinly sliced green beans
1 carrot sliced julienne style
1-2 teaspoons soy sauce
spring water
sesame or olive oil

Heat a stainless steel skillet and add either spring water or a small amount of oil. (You may brush the bottom of the pan with an oil brush.)

Sauté on a medium high to high flame, moving the vegetables in a lively manner in the pan.

Add the vegetables in order from firmest to most delicate, taking care to move the vegetables all the while so they cook evenly.

Sprinkle with a pinch of sea salt or a few drops of soy sauce. Simmer for another 2-3 minutes. Add drops of water if the pan dries out.

Optional step. Add a generous squeeze of fresh ginger juice for a hot taste.

Serve vegetables immediately.

PRESSED SALAD

½ cup sliced cucumbers
½ cup sliced Chinese cabbage
½ cup sliced red radishes
¼ cup sliced celery
¼ cup red onion
1 teaspoon sea salt (1/2 teaspoon per cup of vegetables)

Mix all vegetables with sea salt in a large bowl and gently massage the vegetables until they begin to wilt, turn shiny and release liquid.

Place a dinner plate on top of the vegetables inside the bowl to cover.

Place a weight such as a garden stone, jug of water or sack of beans on top of the plate to exert pressure on the vegetables.

Allow the salad to sit under pressure for 45 minutes to one hour and a half until a significant amount of water is released from the vegetables. Discard the pressing water before serving and *rinse off the vegetables so that they do not taste at all salty.*

DRESSINGS FOR RAW & PRESSED SALADS

Ume-scallion dressing

1 teaspoon umeboshi paste

2 tablespoons finely chopped scallion or chives

¼ cup spring water

Mix all ingredients in a suribachi and pour over fresh blanched vegetables.

Variation. For a richer dressing try adding a teaspoon of tahini or roasted sesame butter. Grated raw onion may be substituted for the scallion.

Miso-lemon-sesame dressing

2 tablespoons toasted sesame seeds

1 teaspoon white or barley miso

2-3 teaspoons fresh lemon juice

¼ cup spring water

Grind the seeds in suribachi until almost fully crushed. Puree the miso in water and add lemon juice. Mix with crushed seeds. Serve over steamed or blanched greens, pressed or fresh salads.

Variation. Tangerine or orange may be substituted for the lemon.

GINGER GREEN BEANS

garlic, minced – can use onion

ginger, grated

green beans

toasted sesame oil

shoyu

Briefly sauté the ginger and onion in the sesame oil. Add the cleaned green beans and sauté until all turn bright green, adding shoyu about a minute before they are done. Stir continuously until all beans are coated.

SWEET SAVORY ONIONS

3 medium onions (cut into thin wedges)

2 cups corn (roughly two ears worth)

1 carrot (cut into match sticks)

2 cloves garlic (pressed or minced) – *optional*

¼ cup chives (minced, for garnish)

2 tablespoons miso

1 tablespoon corn oil

3 tablespoons water

Heat the oil in the wok and sauté garlic and onions for four to five minutes, or until the onions are lightly scorched.

Add carrots and sauté for five minutes.

Dilute miso with water and add to wok.

Add corn and cook for an additional three to four minutes.

Garnish with chives and serve warm.

PICKLE RECIPES
○ ○ ○

QUICK UMEBOSHI PICKLES

½ cup sliced onions

⅓ cup sliced celery

¼ cup sliced cucumbers

⅓ cup umeboshi vinegar

⅔ cup spring water

1 pint sized glass jar

small piece of cheesecloth and rubber band to seal jar

Pack vegetables firmly in jar. Mix umeboshi vinegar and water.

Pour over vegetables to fully cover them. Cover jar with cheesecloth. Leave on kitchen counter overnight or up to 3 days.

Remove from brine, rinse off strong taste and serve.

QUICK SOY SAUCE PICKLES

1 cup onions sliced into ½ moons

⅓ cup soy sauce

⅔ cup water

Slice root or round vegetables ⅛-inch thick. Cover with a mixture of 1 part soy sauce and 2-3 parts water. After 2-3 hours, remove from liquid, rinse if too salty and serve.

SEA VEGETABLES

○ ○ ○

ARAME WITH ONIONS, CORN AND TOFU
1 cup dried, shredded arame
1 cup thinly sliced onions
½ pound fresh tofu
½ cup fresh corn kernels shaved off the cob
spring water

Rinse 1 cup of the arame in a bowl of water. Drain in a colander or strainer until soft.

Layer the onions, corn and arame in a pot. Add enough water to just cover the corn.

Bring to a boil on a medium flame, cover, lower flame. Simmer for 30 minutes. Remove cover and add mashed tofu, and soy sauce to taste.

Simmer for another five minutes until tofu is tender and seasoning has blended in. To cook off remaining liquid, leave cover off.

Mix well before serving.

ARAME WITH ONIONS
one ounce dried arame
equal amount onion
dark sesame oil
soy sauce

Wash and drain one ounce dried arame. Brush a frying pan with dark sesame oil and heat it. Add the onions and sauté for 2-3 minutes (water sauté if oil is to be avoided.)

Place the arame on top of the onions and add enough water to just cover the onions.

Bring to a boil, turn the heat down to low, and add a small amount of shoyu/soy sauce.

Cover and simmer for about 30-35 minutes. Add shoyu to taste (not overly salty).

Simmer for another five to ten minutes, mix and stir until the liquid has evaporated.

Note. Hiziki should be cooked longer, up to 1 ¼-1½ hours total cooking time in order to lose its bitterness and become sweet.

ARAME WITH LOTUS ROOT AND GREEN PEAS

1 cup arame (soaked and rinsed)

1 cup fresh lotus root (thinly sliced and quartered)

1 cup green peas

1 tablespoon sesame oil

2 pinches sea salt

½ to ¾ cup water

Heat the oil in a skillet and sauté the lotus root for 6-7 minutes. Add the sea salt, sauté for another minute then place the arame on top of the lotus root.

Add the water, bring to a boil and simmer 30 minutes without stirring.

SWEET CORN AND ARAME SAUCE

1 cup arame

1 onion, sliced thin

kernels from 2 ears corn

¾-1 cup water

toasted sesame oil

tamari soy sauce

rice vinegar *(optional)*

Wash arame. Place in a pot with water. Bring to a boil and simmer uncovered for 5 minutes.

Lay the onion on top, cover, and simmer 20 minutes. Add more water as needed to keep arame moist but not submerged, you want most of the liquid to be gone when finished cooking.

Add the corn on top (julienne carrot can be substituted), and sprinkle with a few drops of toasted sesame oil. Simmer 10 minutes more.

Season to taste with tamari and vinegar.

BAKED WAKAME WITH ONIONS

2 cups wakame, washed, soaked, and sliced

1-2 cups onions

3-5 tablespoons tahini

1–1 ½ cups water

½ teaspoon ginger juice

¼ cup sesame seeds

tamari

Puree tahini, water and soy sauce, add ginger juice. Mix in onions and wakame.

Place in casserole dish, sprinkle with sesame seeds. Cover and bake 30-35 minutes. Uncover and bake 10 more minutes. May need to add small amount of water during baking if it gets too dry.

LENTIL DINNER WITH WAKAME

6-inch strip wakame

⅓ cup lentils

2 cup short-grain brown rice

1 stalk celery

1 parsnip or carrot

1 onion

fresh rosemary or thyme *(optional)*

2 pinches sea salt

5½ cups water

Cut the wakame in small pieces. Wash the lentils and rice. Cut the vegetables in small compatible shapes.

Layer everything in an oiled baking dish with a tight cover. Add water, bring to a boil on the stovetop, then bake at 375° for 1 hour.

HIZIKI SHIITAKE SIDE DISH

1 cup hiziki

3 cups water

1 medium sliced onion

1 carrot, matchstick sliced

1 tablespoon toasted sesame oil

4 sliced shiitake mushrooms

(if using dried, soak 10 minutes, remove stems, use water)

1 cup apple juice (or ½ cup apple and ½ cup water)

2 tablespoons tamari soy sauce

1 teaspoon fresh grated ginger juice

parsley to garnish

Soak hiziki for 10 minutes in water. Strain and keep soaking water. Sauté onions and carrots in sesame oil until onions are transparent (about 5 minutes).

Add hiziki, shiitake, and soaking water plus 1 cup apple juice to cover surface. Bring to a boil, cover and simmer another 40 minutes to evaporate most of the liquid.

Garnish with parsley and serve hot as a side dish or chilled over a bed of lettuce.

SWEET PARSNIPS AND SEA PALM

1 small onion

2 parsnips

½ cup sea palm (small handful)

½ teaspoon sesame oil

½ cup water (approximately)

½ teaspoon tamari soy sauce, or

1 teaspoon while miso

dash of mirin *(optional)*

Cut onion in half by cutting from end-to-end (not across the middle). Slice in slender half moons.

Cut parsnip in half lengthwise, then slice in long diagonals. Sauté together in oil, stirring for a few minutes until fragrant.

Add sea palm, cut in small pieces, and pour in water. Quickly cover, and simmer 20 minutes. Water should be all gone at the end of cooking.

Season with soy sauce, or miso and mirin.

SIMPLE DESSERTS

○ ○ ○

LEMON PUDDING

2¼ cup plain amasake

1½ cups apple juice

1½ teaspoons grated lemon peel

3 tablespoons agar agar flakes

pinch sea salt

3 heaping tablespoons kuzu

1½ tablespoons lemon juice

1½ teaspoons vanilla *(optional)*

1 tablespoon rice syrup *(optional)*

top with fresh cooked fruit *(optional)*

Heat amasake, juice, agar agar and lemon peel. Simmer 5 minutes until agar dissolves.

Mix kuzu with lemon juice (and add a dash of apple juice until it dissolves). Add to pot and stir until it thickens.

Add salt and vanilla. If too tart, add rice syrup.

Let set for 1 hour in the fridge before serving.

CREAMY RICE PUDDING

1 cup amasake

½ cup water or apple juice

2¼ cups leftover rice

3 tablespoons chopped raisins

3 tablespoons sunflower seeds, or

chopped roasted nuts

1 teaspoon cinnamon, or

grated lemon peel

1 teaspoon vanilla *(optional)*

Combine all the ingredients except vanilla. Heat and simmer with a flame deflector underneath for 10-20 minutes.

APPLESAUCE

4 apples

¼ cup raisins *(optional)*

½ teaspoon cinnamon *(optional)*, or

½ teaspoon minced lemon peel

1 cup water and apple juice (vary mixture to your taste)

1 heaping tablespoon kuzu

1 tablespoon water or juice

Peel, core and slice the apples. Place in saucepan (raisins, cinnamon, or lemon peel) and water. Bring to a boil, cover, and simmer for 10-15 minutes, until apples are tender.

Dissolve kuzu in cold water, add and stir until thick.

For crunch, top with granola, toasted seeds, or nuts.

HOLIDAYS AND PARTIES

o o o

CRANBERRY BRAISED TEMPEH

4 (8 ounce packages) of tempeh

4 cups apple juice

3 cups fresh cranberries

½ teaspoon salt

1½-inch by 4-inch piece of orange peel studded with 4 cloves

¼ cup maple or rice syrup

2 tablespoons tamari or shoyu

2 tablespoons fresh grated ginger

½ teaspoon all spice

½ teaspoon cinnamon

¼ teaspoon each nutmeg and clove

pinch of cayenne

fresh rosemary springs for garnish

This recipe can be done on the stove top. Put all ingredients, including tempeh in a sauce pan and bring to a boil and simmer for 20 to 30 minutes. Serve over brown rice or other whole grain.

STUFFED DELICOTTA SQUASH WITH CRANBERRY CORN BREAD STUFFING

2 good sized squash, halved, seeded and steamed for 10 minutes.

Corn Bread

2½ cup corn meal

1½ cup whole wheat pastry flour

1⅓ cup unbleached white flour

3 tablespoons baking soda

1 teaspoon sea salt

1¼ cup water

1⅓ cup soy milk

⅔ cup olive oil

½ cup rice syrup

½ teaspoon vanilla extract

Mix wet ingredients together. Add dry ingredients and mix until just blended. Pour batter into corn-oiled skillet or pan. Bake 20-25 minutes in preheated 400° oven. Let cool 30 minutes.

Stuffing

1 cup cranberries

1 cup diced celery

1 cup diced onions

½ cup raisins

1 tablespoon corn oil

2 tablespoons shoyu

corn bread, crumbled

Sauté onions for 5 minutes, add celery and sauté 5 more minutes. Add ¼ cup water, cranberries, shoyu and raisins and cover and simmer for 5 minutes.

Add crumbled corn bread and mix thoroughly. Stuff each squash half and bake for 25 minutes at 350°.

STUFFED SQUASH

1 medium-sized Hubbard squash or other hard winter squash of similar size

1 tablespoon corn or sesame oil

1 cup onions, diced

1 cup celery, diced

pinch of sea salt

8 cups whole wheat or whole wheat sourdough bread cubes

(slightly dried out or toasted in a dry skillet until golden brown)

2 cups cooked seitan, cubed

shoyu

1½-2 cups seitan gravy

Carefully cut out a round section of the top of the squash just as would be done for a jack-o-lantern and set it aside. Clean out all the seeds and set aside.

Heat oil in a skillet and sauté the onions for 1-2 minutes. Add the celery and a pinch of salt. Sauté for 1-2 minutes more.

Place this mixture in a large mixing bowl and add the dried or toasted bread cubes and seitan and mix well. Add a small amount of shoyu and mix again.

Stuff the hollowed squash completely full. Pour the seitan gravy over the stuffing and let it seep down.

Place the top back on the squash. Oil the outside skin of the squash with a small amount of sesame oil.

Place the stuffed squash on a baking tray or oven roaster and bake at 325° for about 2 hours.

Remove the top and continue baking for another 25-35 minutes.

To test for doneness, use a shish kebob stick or chopstick to push into the hard skin. When it goes through easily, it is done.

Serve with seitan gravy after scooping out the stuffing and squash for each person.

Variation. Use sautéed vegetables together with cooked brown rice and wild rice; squash and vegetables; millet and vegetables. Add sliced mushrooms, almonds or pine nuts to stuffing.

SOYBEAN SUCCOTASH

16 ounce frozen soybeans (edamame), thawed

3 scallions, sliced diagonally

2 red peppers, diced

2 teaspoons light sesame oil

1¼ cup fresh corn, off the cob, or frozen corn kernels, thawed

pinch of salt

1 teaspoon minced fresh thyme *(optional)*

Prepare soybeans according to package directions; drain and cool. Remove beans from pods; discard the pods.

In large skillet heat oil and over medium-high heat, sauté scallions and red peppers until softened.

Add the corn kernels, salt, minced thyme and soybeans. Cook until thoroughly heated.

TOFU TURKEY

5 pounds tofu, medium firmness

poultry seasoning

herbed whole wheat stuffing

basting liquid

mushroom gravy

parsley or sage for garnish

Poultry Seasoning (makes ½ cup)

¼ cup sage

2 tablespoons marjoram, thyme and savory or rosemary

1 tablespoon celery seed

2 tablespoons black pepper

To prepare homemade poultry seasoning, mix ingredients together well.

Herbed Whole Wheat Stuffing (makes 5 cups)

2 tablespoons sesame oil

1 cup onions, diced

1 cup mushrooms, diced

1 cup celery, diced

2 large cloves garlic, minced

1 tablespoon poultry seasoning

¼ teaspoon sea salt

¼ cup shoyu

4 cups whole wheat bread cut into ½-inch cubes

½ cup parsley chopped

To prepare stuffing, heat oil and sauté onions, mushrooms, celery and garlic. Sprinkle poultry seasoning over vegetables. Dissolve salt in shoyu and add to pot. Stir, cover and continue to cook until vegetables are done, about 5 minutes. Add bread cubes and parsley, mix well.

Basting Liquid

¼–½ cup sesame oil

2 tablespoons – ¼ cup shoyu

Mushroom Gravy (makes 6 cups)

2 tablespoons sesame oil

2 onions, diced

6 cups mushrooms sliced

1 cup whole wheat flour

6–7 cups water

¼ cup shoyu

Mash tofu well. Line a colander (11¾-inch wide including lip) with a single layer of moistened cheesecloth. Transfer tofu to colander.

Press tofu to flatten and fold edges of cheesecloth over it. Place a cake tin or other flat object over the surface of the tofu and weight it down with a heavy object (about 5 pounds) to press liquid from tofu for 1 hour.

Hollow out tofu within one inch of colander. Pack in stuffing and cover with remaining tofu. Pat down so surface is flat and firm.

Oil a baking sheet and flip filled tofu onto sheet so the flat surface faces down. Remove cheesecloth.

Mix basting liquid and brush tofu with it. Cover tofu with foil. Bake at 400° for 1 hour.

Remove foil and baste. Return to oven to bake uncovered until "skin" become golden brown, about 1 hour more. Baste again halfway through.

PAN CORNBREAD

2½ cups corn meal

1½ cups whole wheat pastry flour

1½ cups unbleached white flour

3 tablespoons baking powder

1 teaspoon salt

1½ cups water

1¼ cups soy milk

⅔ cup olive oil

½ cup pure maple syrup

½ teaspoon pure vanilla extract

Preheat oven to 400°. Oil a 9"x12" baking pan with the olive oil.

In a large bowl, mix together all of the dry ingredients.

In separate bowl, stir together all of the wet ingredients.

Add wet mix to dry ingredients and mix together until blended.

Pour batter into the pan, bake 20-25 minutes, or until a tester in the center comes out clean.

Let cool for 30 minutes on a wire rack. Cut into squares and serve.

VEGETABLE DUMPLING
Pre-made dumpling skins
1 onion, sliced to half moons
¼ head cabbage, shredded
2 carrots, grated
1/3 package arame, soaked 10 minutes and chopped
½ bunch collard greens or bok choy, sliced thin
toasted sesame oil

Dipping Sauce
shoyu
ginger juice

Sauté onions in sesame oil several minutes.

Add all other vegetables and greens. Sauté several minutes.

Sprinkle shoyu on everything. Simmer 5 minutes.

Squeeze ginger juice. Add chopped scallions. Let sauté cool.

Put 1 teaspoon filling in dumplings. Wet skin around edge and pinch closed. Pan fry, in oil or water, until golden.

WALDORF SALAD

¼ cup toasted walnuts

¼ cup raisins

2 cups apples, diced

2 ribs of celery, diced

1 grated carrot

2 tablespoons of dulse flakes, or soaked pieces of dulse sliced and cut up

(smoked dulse is especially nice)

½ cup Veganaise (without cane sugar) or use tofu mayonnaise recipe *(listed in bean recipes)*

1 teaspoon umeboshi vinegar

Put everything together in bowl and mix in a small amount veganaise and splash in some umeboshi vinegar. Taste and season to your liking.

MILLET "MASHED POTATOES"

2 cups millet

1 small cauliflower (approximately 2 cups flowerettes)

¼ teaspoon sea salt

7 cups water

extra water for mashing

Light roast millet.

Bring water to a boil, add millet, cauliflower and salt. Cover and simmer 25 minutes.

Puree in a food mill or food processor, adding a little water if necessary.

BROWN GRAVY

6 tablespoons whole wheat flour

2 tablespoons sesame oil

½ onion, minced fine, or

6 mushrooms, sliced

2 cups water or vegetable stock

1 teaspoon thyme

2 teaspoons marjoram

1-2 tablespoons tamari soy sauce

½ teaspoon minced lemon peel *(optional)*

Roast the flour by stirring in a skillet over medium heat until fragrant, but not browned.

In a saucepan, sauté onion or mushroom in oil. Add flour, cook 5 minutes on low heat, stirring occasionally.

Briskly stir in water. Add herbs and tamari.

Put a flame spreader under the pot, cover, and simmer 20 minutes. Adjust seasoning to taste.

CAESAR SALAD

Dressing

2 tablespoons blanched almonds

3 cloves garlic, minced

2 tablespoons Dijon mustard

3 tablespoons nutritional yeast

2 tablespoons soy sauce

3 tablespoons fresh lemon juice

¼ cup water

1 tablespoon olive oil

Combine all ingredients in a food processor.

Croutons

3-4 slices whole wheat sourdough bread, trimmed and cubed

olive oil

½ teaspoon each rosemary, marjoram, garlic powder, sea salt

Fry bread in oil and herbs. For crunchier croutons bake for 5-10 minutes.

Dress 1 large head romaine with dressing, add croutons.

LINZER TORT COOKIE

1 cup ground almonds, hazelnuts or macadamia nuts

1 cup whole wheat pastry flour

1 cup ground oats

½ cup corn or olive oil

½ cup rice syrup or ½ cup rice syrup and ¼ cup maple syrup

¼ teaspoon cinnamon

pinch sea salt

1 jar raspberry jam, non-sweetened

Mix dry ingredients. Mix wet ingredients. Combine wet ingredients with dry and mix.

Form dough into balls, make indentation for jam. Put in jam. Bake 350° for 10-15 minutes.

APPLE PIE CRUST

(with filling and whipped cream)

3 cups whole wheat pastry flour

½-⅔ cup olive oil

½ teaspoon sea salt

spring water

Preheat oven to 375°. Sift the flour and sea salt into a large bowl. Add the oil and mix through the flour to resemble breadcrumbs.

Add enough flour to form a dough. Handle the dough as little as possible to keep it light and flaky. Place the dough in the freezer for about 5 minutes.

Roll out the pastry and place in a pie dish that has been lightly oiled. Place in the oven and bake for 15 minutes. Remove and turn the oven heat down to 350°.

Let the pie shell cool before adding the apples. Any leftover pastry can be rolled out and cut into shapes with a pastry cutter. Use to decorate the top of the pie.

Filling

10 medium apples washed, peeled and sliced

2-3 cups apple juice

pinch sea salt

1 tablespoon rice syrup

2 tablespoons kuzu diluted in ½ cup cold spring water

Place the apples, apple juice and sea salt in a pot. Bring to a boil on a medium flame. Simmer for about 10 minutes or until soft.

Remove the apples and place in the pie shell. Add the diluted kuzu and rice malt to the apple juice. Stir gently until thick. Pour over the top of the apples.

Arrange the pastry shapes over the apples. Bake the pie at 350° for 35 minutes. Remove and allow to cool before serving.

Tofu Whipped Cream

1 cake tofu, firm

2 tablespoons tahini

1 tablespoon vanilla

6 tablespoons rice syrup

Chill for ½ to 1 hour before using.

APPLE-BLUEBERRY CRISP

6 apples

1-quart blueberries, washed and clean

4 cups apple juice

6 tablespoons arrow root or kuzu

1 teaspoon vanilla

pinch sea salt

Topping

3 cups oats

2 cups barley flour

¾ cup olive oil

¾ cup rice syrup

1 cup chopped walnuts or pecans

¼ teaspoon sea salt

¼ teaspoon cinnamon

Slice apples and place them in a 9"x12" baking pan with blueberries.

Heat apple juice, add dissolved arrowroot (can dissolve in some of the cold apple juice). Bring to boil and let simmer. Turn off heat and add vanilla.

Dry roast the oats and barley flour. Heat oil and syrup together, pour over flour mixture. Add nuts and cinnamon.

Pour apple juice mixture over apples and blueberries. Cover with topping-oat mixture. Cover and bake in preheated 350° oven 30 minutes.

Uncover and bake 10-20 minutes.

SPECIAL REMEDIES
○ ○ ○

SWEET VEGETABLE DRINK

½ cup onions

½ cup carrots

½ cup round, green cabbage

½ cup sweet winter squash

4-5 cups spring water

Finely chop all vegetables into small pieces. Bring the spring water to a boil. (Use 3 times the amount of water to vegetables.)

Add vegetables to the boiling water, leave the pot uncovered until it returns to a boil.

Cover the pot, reduce the flame to low and simmer 20 minutes. Strain out the vegetables and discard them. Drink the broth warm or hot.

CARROT-DAIKON DRINK

¼-½ cup fresh grated carrot

¼-½ cup fresh grated daikon

1 cup spring water

Couple drops shoyu

Place carrot, daikon and water in saucepan. Bring to a boil, then lower the flame. Simmer 3-4 minutes.

Add the drops of shoyu and any other specified ingredient. Eat and drink the vegetables and the broth.

LEAFY GREENS JUICE

Benefit: Helps dissolve heavy, stagnated protein and fat. Nourishes the liver.

1 cup finely sliced leafy greens such as kale, collards, dandelion, daikon or turnip leaves,
Chinese cabbage or bok choy
2 cups spring water
pinch sea salt or drop of soy sauce

Place greens and water in saucepan and bring to a boil. Simmer uncovered
2-3 minutes.

Add the pinch of sea salt or drop soy sauce and mix gently. Drink hot or
at room temperature.

UME-SHO-BANCHA

*Benefit: Strengthens/alkalizes the blood, regulates digestion and circulation, relieves fatigue and
weakness.*

½-1 umeboshi plum
several drops to ½-1 teaspoon soy sauce
1 cup hot kukicha twig tea

Place umeboshi and soy sauce in the bottom of a tea cup. Pour the hot
twig tea on top of the plum and shoyu.

Stir gently and drink immediately. Eat the plum along with the tea.

UME-SHO-KUZU

Benefit: Strengthens intestines, kidneys, promotes good digestion, restores energy.

1 heaping teaspoon kuzu powder
½-1 umeboshi plum
several drops soy sauce
1 cup, plus 2 tablespoons, cold spring water

Dissolve the kuzu powder in 2 tablespoons cold water. Add this to a saucepan with the remainder of the spring water. Add the crushed umeboshi plum.

Bring the mixture to a boil, reduce the heat to a simmer. Stir constantly until the liquid becomes transparent and thick.

ADUKI BEAN TEA

Benefit: Regulates kidney and urinary tract function, promotes smooth bowel movements.

1 cup aduki beans
½-1 inch strip (dry) kombu
4 cups spring water

Place ingredients in pan and bring to a boil.
Cover, reduce flame and simmer 30 minutes or longer.
Strain and drink the tea hot.
Cook the beans with additional water until soft and edible.

BLACK SOYBEAN TEA

Benefit: Warms the body, smooths the bowel movement, relaxes a tight chest, reduces coughs, nourishes female sexual organs.

1 cup black soybeans, washed
4 cups spring water
pinch sea salt

Place ingredients in a pot and bring to a boil. Reduce flame and simmer 30-45 minutes. Add a few grains sea salt, simmer 5 more minutes.

Strain and drink hot. Your may continue to cook the beans until they are edible. Use additional water and seasoning.

FRESH LOTUS ROOT TEA

Benefit: Dissolve excess mucus in the respiratory system, eases cough.

½ cup juices squeezed from 1 cup fresh grated lotus root
½ cup spring water
pinch sea salt

To grate lotus root, wash it well and use a flat grater to obtain a juicy pulp. Squeeze out juice with bare hands into a cup or bowl or squeeze through cheesecloth.

Place lotus juice, water and sea salt in a saucepan and bring slowly to a boil, stirring continuously.

Reduce the flame to low and simmer 2-3 minutes. Drink immediately while hot.

MENU PLANS

MENU PLANS

∘ ∘ ∘

WEEK ONE

	MONDAY	TUESDAY	WEDNESDAY	THURSDAY	FRIDAY	SATURDAY	SUNDAY
BREAKFAST	Soft Rice Blanched Kale Miso Soup	Pan Fried Mochi Steamed Bok Choy Miso Soup	Soft Rice with Barley Sauteed Cabbage Miso Soup	Soft Rice *(use leftover grain)* Blanched Kale Miso Soup	Whole Oats Porridge with Raisins Miso Soup	**BRUNCH** Miso Vegetable Soft Rice *(leftover)* Porridge with Toasted Pumpkin Seeds	Soft Polenta Blanched Collard Greens Miso Soup
SNACK	Steamed Cauliflower	leftover Carrots and Tops	Cabbage *(from breakfast)*	leftover Minestrone Soup	leftover nishime	Tempeh with Sauerkraut and Onions Steamed Broccoli	leftovers from Saturday
LUNCH	Quinoa Tempeh Tuna Salad Hiziki Shiitake Dish Pressed Salad	Sushi with carrot, red cabbage and cucumber *(can use leftover rice)* leftover Split Pea Soup Blanched Greens Pressed Salad	Grain Patties with mustard and sauerkraut *(use leftover rice with chickpeas)* Blanched Collard Greens leftover Kinpira Applesauce leftover sushi	Millet Mashed Potatoes with Gravy leftover Squash Azuki Beans and Chestnuts Blanched Greens Pressed Salad with leftover ume scallion dressing	Grain Salad *(use leftover rice with black soybeans)* leftover quick sauteed vegetables Natto Condiment Pressed Salad	Pressed Salad	
SNACK	leftovers from lunch	leftover sushi	leftover grain pattie	leftover greens	leftover grain salad	leftover kinpira	
DINNER	Pressure Cooked Rice Steamed Carrots and Tops Dried Daikon Radish with Vegetables and Kombu Split Pea Soup Pickle	Rice with Chickpeas Sauteed Greens Kinpira Squash and Carrot Ginger Soup Pickle	Boiled Rice Squash Azuki Beans and Chestnuts Blanched Greens with Ume Scallion Dressing Minestrone Soup Pressed Salad	Rice w/ Black Soybeans Quick Sauteed Vegetables Nishime Cream of Broccoli Soup Pressed Salad	Boiled Rice Arame with Onions, Corn and Tofu Kinpira Parsnip Soup Pickle	Lentil Dinner with Wakame Boiled Salad with Miso Lemon Sesame Dressing Pickle	Rice with Wild Rice Steamed Haddock Ginger Green Beans Nishime Hot and Sour Soup Apple Pie with Tofu Whipped Cream

	MONDAY	TUESDAY	WEDNESDAY	THURSDAY	FRIDAY	SATURDAY	SUNDAY
BREAKFAST	Soft Rice with Wheatberries and Apple Blanched Kale Miso Soup with Tofu	Soft Polenta Boiled Salad Miso Soup	Leftover soft rice Steamed Cabbage and Cauliflower Miso Soup	Miso Vegetable Soft Millet Porridge with Toasted Pumpkin Seeds Blanched Kale	Whole Oat Porridge Sauteed Cabbage with Sauerkraut Miso Soup	**BRUNCH** Mochi Waffles with Raspberry Sauce Nabe Style Vegetables and Tofu Pickle	Soft Rice with Rye *(use left-over grain)* Steamed Greens *(Cabbage and Bok Choy)* Miso Soup
SNACK	leftover kale	leftover steamed daikon and tops	leftover kinpira	Lightly Steamed Vegetables Soup	leftover mushroom barley soup		
LUNCH	Millet Mashed Potatoes with Gravy Lightly Stewed Vegetables with Seitan Blanched Collard Greens Pressed Salad	Grain Salad *(use leftover rice with azuki beans)* Nishime Pickle *(sauerkraut)* Lemon Pudding	Scrambled Tofu with Vegetables Blanched Mustard Greens with leftover miso dressing leftover black bean soup Pressed Salad	Burritos (with leftover rice & pinto beans) leftover Carrots and Tops Blanched Greens Pickle leftover greens	Quinoa Salad with Sunflower Seeds leftover arame Tempeh with Sauerkraut and Onion Pressed Salad leftover grain salad		leftovers from Saturday
SNACK	leftover millet and stewed vegetables	leftover nishime	leftover scrambled tofu with vegetables	leftover Blanched Kale	leftover Quinoa Salad with sunflower seeds	leftover nabe vegetables	
DINNER	Pressure Cooked Rice with Azuki Beans Steamed Daikon and Tops Baked Wakame with Onions Corn Chowdah Pickle	Pressure Cooked Rice Blanched Greens with Miso Orange Sesame Dressing Kinpira Black Bean Soup Pressed Salad	Boiled Rice Sweet and Sour Pinto Beans Steamed Carrots and Tops Noodles in Broth Pickle	Mushroom Barley Soup Arame with Lotus Root and Green Peas Nishime Pressed Salad	Pressure Cooked Rice Lightly Stewed Vegetables Sweet Savory Onions Black Soybean Stew Pickle	Boiled Rice with Rye Nishime Miso Soup Pressed Salad	Rice with Wild Rice Steamed Cod Kinpira Caesar Salad Pickle Apple Blueberry Crisp

WEEK THREE

∘ ∘ ∘

	MONDAY	TUESDAY	WEDNESDAY	THURSDAY	FRIDAY	SATURDAY	SUNDAY
BREAKFAST							
	Pan Fried Mochi Steamed Watercress and Bok Choy Miso Soup	Soft Rice with Corn *(use left-over grain)* Blanched Kale Miso Soup	Soft Rice *(use leftover grain)* Sauteed Greens Miso Soup	Soft Polenta Quick Sauteed Vegetables Miso Soup	Miso Vegetable Soft Grain Porridge *(use leftover rice with barley)* with toasted pumpkin seeds	**BRUNCH** Pasta Salad with Seitan *(use leftover noodles)* Quick Sauteed Vegetables Pressed Salad	Whole Oats Porridge with raisins Blanched Greens Miso Soup
SNACK							
	leftover grain from breakfast	leftover boiled salad	leftover hiziki shiitake dish	leftover sauteed vegetables	leftover kinpira		leftovers from Saturday
LUNCH							
	Rice with Corn Tempeh Tuna Salad Quick Sauteed Vegetables Pressed Salad	leftover lentil dinner Sauteed Greens Pressed Salad	Chickpea Burgers on Steamed Bread with Sauerkraut leftover roots and tops Steamed Greens Creamy Rice Pudding	Grain Salad *(use leftover rice with black soybeans)* Nishime Pressed Salad leftover Blanched Kale	Boiled Rice Scrambled Tofu with Vegetables leftover green beans Pressed Salad		
SNACK							
	leftover tempeh tuna salad	Steamed Broccoli & Cauliflower with leftover sesame dressing	leftover chickpea burger	leftover grain salad	Steamed Vegetables	leftover pasta salad	
DINNER							
	Lentil Dinner with Wakame Boiled Salad with Sesame Dressing Pickle	Millet Sweet Vegetable Soup Hiziki Shiitake Dish Steamed Turnips and Tops Chickpeas Pickle	Rice with Black Soybeans Dried Daikon Radish with Vegetables and Kombu Squash and Carrot Ginger Soup Pressed Salad	Pressure Cooked Rice with Barley Ginger Green Beans Azuki Bean Vegetable Soup Kinpira Pickle	Rice Balls Sweet Parsnips and Sea Palm Baked Kidney Beans with Miso and Apple Butter Broccoli Noodle Soup Pickle	Jessica's Hamburger Helper Blanched Greens Pickle	Boiled Rice Steamed Red Snapper Sweet Savory Onions Lentil Soup Pickle *(sauerkraut)* Linzer Tort Cookies

WEEK FOUR
∘ ∘ ∘

	MONDAY	TUESDAY	WEDNESDAY	THURSDAY	FRIDAY	SATURDAY	SUNDAY
BREAKFAST	Whole Oat Porridge with Apples Blanched Greens	Miso Vegetable Soft Rice and Barley *(use leftover grain)* *Porridge* Sauteed Mizuna	Soft Rice *(use leftover grain)* Blanched Kale Miso Soup	Soft Polenta Quick Sauteed Vegetables Miso Soup	Soft Polenta Quick Steamed Greens Miso Soup	**BRUNCH** Mochi Waffles with Blueberry Sauce Nabe Style Vegetables with Tofu	Miso Vegetable Soft Rice *(use leftover grain)* Porridge with Toasted Pumpkin Seeds Quick Sauteed Greens
SNACK	leftover blanched greens	leftover Turnips and Tops	leftover hiziki shiitake dish	leftover blanched kale	leftover noodles in broth	Waldorf Salad	
LUNCH	Pressure Cooked Rice with Black Soybeans Lightly Steamed Vegetables with Ume Scallion Dressing Pressed Salad	Grain Salad *(use leftover grain)* Nishime Pressed Salad	Chickpea Burgers on Steamed Bread with Sauerkraut leftover roots and tops Steamed Greens Creamy Rice Pudding	Hummus Wrap *(use leftover chickpeas)* Cucumber Pressed Salad Lemon Pudding	Millet with Sweet Vegetables Blanched Mustard Greens with Sesame Dressing Baked Wakame with Onions		leftovers from Saturday
SNACK	leftover steamed vegetables	leftover nishime	leftover chickpea burger	leftover carrot and cucumber pressed salad with hummus	leftover mustard greens with sesame dressing	Pan Fried Rice with Millet Patties *(use leftover grain)*	
DINNER	Pressure Cooked Rice with Barley Steamed Turnips and Tops Lightly Stewed Vegetables with Tempeh Cream of Broccoli Soup Pickle	Boiled Rice Arame with Lotus Root and Green Peas Gingered Chickpeas Squash and Carrot Ginger Soup Pickle	Rice with Black Soybeans Dried Daikon Radish with Vegetables and Kombu Squash and Carrot Ginger Soup Pressed Salad	Noodles in Broth Lightly Stewed Vegetables with Dried Tofu Boiled Salad Pickle	Pressure Cooked Rice Squash Azuki Beans and Chestnuts Steamed Daikon and Tops Pickle	Boiled Rice Blanched Greens Dried Daikon Radish with Vegetables and Kombu Nishime Pickle	Pressure Cooked Rice with Wheatberries Quick Sauteed Vegetables Arame with Onions, Corn and Tofu Fish Stew Apple Pie

RECOMMENDED READING:

The China Study, Dr. T. Colin Campbell and Thomas M. Campbell, II

The Macrobiotic Way, Michio Kushi
The Macrobiotic Approach to Cancer, Michio Kushi
Diet for a Strong Heart, Michio Kushi with Alex Jack
The Macrobiotic Path to Total Health, Michio Kushi with Alex Jack
Hypoglycemia and Diabetes, Aveline Kushi
Crime and Diet, Michio Kushi

Nature's Cancer Fighting Foods, Verne Varona

The Self-Healing Cookbook, Kristina Turner

The Food Revolution, John Robbins
Diet for a New America, John Robbins

Zen Macrobiotics for Americans, Roger Mason

Molecules of Emotion, Candace Pert, Ph.D.

Awakening Your Intuition, Mona Lisa Schultz, MD.

Unfolding, Julia Mossbridge

Living in the Light, Shakti Gawain

Greens and Grains on the Deep Blue Sea Cookbook:
    Fabulous Vegetarian Cuisine from the Taste of Health Cruises,
    Sandy Pukel and Mark Hanna

Life's Delicate Balance: The Causes and Prevention of Breast Cancer,
    Janette Sherman, MD.

Prepare for Surgery, Heal Faster, Peggy Huddleston, RN

Stand Up For Your Life, Cheryl Richardson

*Nagasaki 1945: The First Full-Length Eyewitness Account of the
    Atomic Bomb Attack on Nagasaki*, Tatsuichiro Akizuki

Amazing Grains, by Joanne Saltzman

*Positive Energy Practices, How to Attract Uplifting People
    and Combat Energy Vampires*, Judith Orloff, MD

Don't Drink Your Milk, Frank A. Oski, MD

Ten Steps to Strengthening Health, Denny Waxman and Ruth Ann Flynn
Strengthening Health Publications, Philadelphia, PA. (215) 732-2331

American Macrobiotic Cuisine, Meredith McCarty

*The Crazy Makers, How the Food Industry is Destroting Our Brains
and Harming Our Children*, Carol Simontacchi

*Addictive Foods, Reversing Diabetes, Food for Life, Breaking the Food Seduction,
Eat Right & Life Longer, Foods That Cause You to Lose Weight*, Neal Barnard, MD

The Hip Chick's Guide to Macrobiotics, Jessica Porter

Because I Can, Joan Borgatti,www.coachborgatti.com

The Joy Diet, Finding Your Own North Star, Martha Beck, Ph. D

Healing Your Family House, 5 Steps to Break Free of Destructive Patterns,
Rebecca Linder Hintze

Love, Medicine, and Miracles, Bernie Siegel, MD

MACROBIOTIC RECOVERY STORIES:

My Beautiful Life, Mina Dobic, Ph.D. (ovarian cancer)

When Hope Never Dies, Marlene McKenna (malignant melanoma)

Recovery from Cancer, Elaine Nussbaum (ovarian cancer)

Kamikaze Cowboy, Dirk Benedict (prostate cancer)

Healing Miracles from Macrobiotics,
Dr. Jean Kohler and Mary Alice Kohler (pancreatic cancer)

Macrobiotic Miracle: How a Vermont Family Overcame Cancer
Virginia Brown and Susan Stayman (malignant melanoma)

Cancer-Free, Kit Kitatani (stomach cancer)

Controlling Crohn's Disease The Natural Way, Virginia Harper (Crohn's disease)

AUDIO CD'S:

Self Esteem, Caroline Myss

Positive Healing, Judith Orloff, MD.

Healing Music of Zimbabwe, Erica Azim, The Relaxation Company
Dandemutande-a resource for Zimbabwe, 122
E. Pike St.,#1163, Seattle, WA 98122-3934, USA, Email: dandemutande.org

Honoring Our Breasts: A Guided Self-Exam to Music
Dr. Dixie Mills

RECOMMENDED WEBSITES:

www.megwolff.com: My personal website where you can find my current events (including lectures, book signings and cooking classes) along with other macrobiotic survivor stories and many other resources to help you on your path to health.

www.macrobreastcancersurvivors.com: My website presents many breast cancer survivor's stories as well as other recovery stories. It provides information and support to survivors and those currently recovering from breast cancer, as well as their families and friends. The focus is on macrobiotics as a way of life and alternative or additional means of recovery.

www.kushiinstitute.org: a non-profit organization in Becket, Massachusetts that teaches macrobiotic cooking and lifestyle.

www.pcrm.org: Physicians Committee for Responsible Medicine (PCRM) was founded in 1985. It is a nonprofit organization that promotes preventive medicine, good nutrition, and clinical research, and it encourages higher standards for ethics and effectiveness in research.

www.organicconsumers.org: This website is hosted by the Organic Consumers Association. They advocate the labeling of genetically engineered food and promote organic food and sustainable agriculture.

www.amberwaves.org: A website dedicated to a campaign to save organic rice and wheat from the hazards of genetic engineering.

www.whollymacrobiotics.com: Gayle Stolove, RN and breast cancer survivor.

www.drdixiemills.com: Dixie J. Mills, MD, FACS is a Harvard-trained general surgeon who has been specializing in breast care since 1989. Her website offers breast cancer stories and resources and features her CD *Honoring Our Breast: A Guided Self Exam to Music.*

www.drnorthrup.com: Dr. Christiane Northrup helps you to engage in your own inner wisdom. Her site features upcoming events, daily inspiration, health & energy centers and a newsletter.

AMPUTEE WEBSITES:

www.amputee-coalition.org: The ACA Amputee Coalition of America's mission is to reach out to people with limb loss and to empower them through education, support and advocacy.

www.ertlreconstruction.com: The mission of Ertl Reconstruction is to provide accurate information about the Ertl Procedure and the resources that are available for both the layperson and the medical community.

www.oandp.com/resources/organizations/barr/index2.htm: The Barr Foundation

MACROBIOTIC VACATIONS

atasteofhealth.org: Holistic cruise vacations with some of the world's leading authorities and experts in holistic living and natural heath. Hosted by Sandy Pukel and Mark Hanna.

christinacooks.com: Healthy vacations to exotic locations lead by Christina Pirello (past trips include Belize, Barbados, Italy, Puerta Vallarta, Mexico).

THE KUSHI INSTITUTE

The leading macrobiotic educational center in the world. Students from around the globe attend residential-style programs on the macrobiotic approach to health and healing.

P.O. Box 16

Becket, MA 01223-0007

Phone: 1-800-975-8744

www.kushiinstitute.org

THE KUSHI INSTITUTE OF EUROPE

Weteringschans 65

1017 RX Amsterdam, RX

Phone: +31 (0) 20 625 75 13

Fax: +31 (0) 20 622 73 20

Email: kushi@macrobiotics.nl

MICHIO KUSHI

Founder of the Kushi Institute and the One Peaceful World Society, Author, Lecturer

P.O. Box 16

Becket, MA 01223-0007

Email: info@michiokushi.org

www.michiokushi.org

LUCHI & NAOKI BARANDA

Kushi Institute Instructors/Senior Macrobiotic Counselors

P.O. Box 16

Becket, MA 01223

DEBORAH WRIGHT

Breast Cancer Survivor

Kushi Institute

P.O. Box 16

Becket, MA 01223

BETTINA ZUMDICK

A Kushi Institute Instructor, counselor and interfaith minister

Kushi Institute

P.O. Box 16

Becket, MA 01223

JAMES CAOLA

Philadelphia, PA

James Caola is a macrobiotic chef, writer and teacher in Philadelphia, Pennsylvania. He began the study and practice of macrobiotic philosophy and cooking in 1986, with an educational background in the social sciences, art and music. He began studies in macrobiotics at a Way Of Life seminar conducted by Denny Waxman at the now defunct East West Center of Philadelphia. He has also studied the writings of George Oshawa, Michio Kushi, Herman Aihara, Naboru Muramoto and other well known writers on macrobiotic philosophy and cooking.

His website supports the practice of macrobiotics. The site is found at www.geocities.com/gur2 and includes basic macrobiotic principles, hundreds of recipes, cooking techniques, menu models, bibliography, links to other macrobiotic sites, and reprints of articles by Mr. Caola originally appearing in MacroChef, Christina Cooks Magazine, or Christina's Living Healthy Journal. Anyone interested in Mr. Caola's cooking or instruction services can contact him at (215) 339-5233.

PREVENTIVE MEDICINE CENTER

1000 Asylum Avenue, #2109

Hartford, CT 06105

Phone: (860) 549-3444 or (800) 789-PREV

www.prevmedctr.org

The PMC is a 501(c)(3) non-profit charitable and tax deductible organization that provides resources and information on conventional, alternative, and complementary medicines, advice on whole foods/high fiber approaches to healthful nutrition including macrobiotics, cooking classes, and lectures.

The Preventive Medicine Center is dedicated to promoting a realistic, supportive, holistic approach to health—achieving disease prevention and reversal, where possible, through a combination of innovative, traditional, and alternative methods.

H. ROBERT SILVERSTEIN, M.D.

Fellow of the American College of Cardiology

Fellow of the American College of Preventive Medicine

Medical Director of the Preventative Medical Center (above)

BONNIE KRAMER

Director of Nutritional Services of the Preventative Medical Center (above)

Phone: (860) 489-6186.

Bonnie has been the Director of Nutritional Services since 1995 and she has cooked and lectured at several area hospitals and has appeared on numerous TV and radio shows in Connecticut and Massachusetts.

The Preventive Medicine Center provides macrobiotic cooking classes and a lecture series during the fall and spring. Bonnie, who studied at the Kushi Institute, is one of the instructors for the cooking classes.

For those who do not have the time to cook, she also prepares and delivers complete meals, from soup to dessert, three times a week (Monday, Wednesday, & Thursday).

STACEY L. ADKINS, MD.

Stacey L. Adkins, MD. practices macrobiotic counseling and teaches cooking classes in both Washington, DC. and New York City. She has studied macrobiotics extensively over the past nine years with Denny Waxman, a renowned macrobiotic counselor and educator and Director of the Strengthening Health Institute. Dr. Adkins completed the Macrobiotic Counselor Training Program at the Strengthening Health Institute and is now engaged in the Graduate Studies Program, as well as being on the Board of Directors of the school. She also completed the Counselor Training Program at the Vega Institute and has studied with Michio Kushi in his Advanced Training Seminars.

Dr. Adkins received her MD from Stanford University, followed by residency training in Internal Medicine and Anesthesiology at the University of Pennsylvania. She completed a clinical fellowship in Cardiac Anesthesiology at New York University and a research fellowship in Neuroscience at the University of California at San Diego. She has held faculty positions at NYU, UCSD and the Medical College of Pennsylvania.

PHIL & YUKIKO JANNETTA, DIRECTORS

Macrobiotics of Western PA

Personal consultations, workshops and seminars, cooking classes
    and Palm Healing sessions.

Email: philjannetta@hotmail.com

Phone: (412) 782-5762

Phil was certified in 1980 by Michio & Aveline Kushi as a Macrobiotic Teacher and Counselor. Yukiko studied macrobiotics and cooking while living at the Kushi house in Boston and graduated from Lima Ohsawa's Cooking Program in Tokyo.

SUSAN & JEREMY HIGA

Macrobiotic counselors and cooking teachers; lecturers with a focus on strong families

P.O. Box 638

Great Barrington, MA 01230

KATIE POWER

Stratton, VT

Phone: (540) 846-2198

Cell: (239) 770-6335

WARREN KRAMER

28 Pertshire Road #2

Brighton, MA 02135

Phone: (617) 562-1110

Email: warrenkramer@verizon.net

www.macrobioticsnewengland.com

Counselor, cooking teacher, lecturer. Warren's school, Macrobiotics of New England, offers cooking classes and lectures, health counseling, and a monthly community dinner. Visit his website for event listings.

Warren is also a facutly member of the Kushi Institute, Strengthening Health Institute and the New England School of Acupuncture. Member of the Macrobiotic Educator's Association. U.S. and international travel.

DOROTHY ROGERS

Boston Center for Natural Living

124 Pleasant Street

Winthrop, MA 02152

Phone: (617) 539-0006

Shiatsu Practitioner, Macrobiotic Counselor, Macrobiotic Cooking Instructor

CARRY WOLF

MEA Health Education & Cooking Instructor

Holistic Education

Natural Health & Lifestyle Counseling

Classes – Lectures – Seminars

Available Internationally

Phone: (413) 623-5810

MICHAEL ROSSOFF, L.AC.

Asheville, NC.

Michael has practiced macrobiotics since 1969. Since the mid-1970's, Michael has taught and counseled on macrobiotics and natural healing. Previous publisher of MacroMuse magazine, Michael has taught throughout the USA, plus Canada, England, Switzerland, Italy and Israel. He has practiced acupuncture since 1978 and was academic dean of Atlantic University of Chinese Medicine for 3 years. He lives in Asheville, NC, where he does acupuncture, teaching and personal counseling.

Phone: (828) 258-1883

www.michaelrossoff.com

LINO STANCHICH

Senior Certified Macrobiotic Counselor

Licensed Nutritionist, Lincensed Bodywork Therapist

Educator, Author

101 Willow Lake Drive

Asheville, NC 28805

www.macrobioticconsultation.com

Books: *Power Eating Program, You Are How You Eat, Macrobiotic Healing Secrets*

ELLEN THOMAS

New York City, NY

Macrobiotic and Vegetarian Chef

Five years of experience, trained at Kushi Institute,

serving New York City and surrounding areas.

Phone: (678) 592-8820

JEANNE COOPER

Jeanne teaches introductory classes in macrobiotics in a

small group setting of 5-10 people.

302 Berwick Court

Wake Forest, NC 27587

Phone: (919) 556-4538

ROSEMARY TRAILL

Macorbiotic Counselor and Cooking Instructor

Pittsburgh, PA

Email: macrorose@msn.com

VIRGINIA M. HARPER

Counselor/School/Author

Franklin, Tennessee

The Ki of Life Learning Center has supported the Greater Nashville Macrobiotic
Community by providing a central location for macrobiotic & nutrition related events .
www.kioflife.com

GALE & ALEX JACK

This site offers information on macrobiotics and personal counseling services

www.macrobioticpath.com

Beckett, MA

JOHN KOZINSKI, MEA

Senior Macrobiotic Counselor

30 years counseling seriously ill and healthy lifestyle seekers using modern approaches including diet/complementary modalities.

Phone: (413) 623-5925

www.macrobiotic.com

JUDITH D. MACKENNEY, D.C.ED.

(Dr. of C.O.R.E. Education)

Certified Holistic Health Counselor (CHC)

      & Member of the American Society of Alternative Therapists

Macrobiotic Counselor

Member of the Faculty & Life Guidance Department & Way To Health Program

A Macrobiotic Survivor/Thriver of Non-Hodgkins Nodular Lymphoma

Stage IV cancer diagnosed in 1991

HARMONY HAVEN HEALING ARTS

712 Quail Court

Nokomis

Sarasota County, FL 34275-2542

Phone: (941) 488-9509

ANTONIA DEMAS, PH.D

Director of the Food Studies Institute

60 Cayuga Street

Trumansburg, NY 14886

Phone: (607) 387-6884

Email: antonia8@yahoo.com

www.foodstudies.org

DENNY WAXMAN

Teacher, counselor, and writer on health, natural healing and macrobiotics.

Philadelphia, PA

Phone: 215.271.1858

www.dennywaxman.com

His school, The Strengthening Health Institute (www.strenthening health.org) was founded in 1997 to teach others how to create lasting health and how to discover and live fully their life's dream.

WILLIAM (BILL) AND CAROL TIMS, ND, PH.D.

Senior Macrobiotic Consultants—25 years

Bill is the former Vice President East West Foundation and Kushi Institute Instructor

Both Bill and Carol can be reached through The Natural Health Center (listed below).

THE NATURAL HEALTH CENTER

Offering private Macrobiotic Counseling and German Vega Bio-Testing

45 N. Hartman Ave.

Fayetteville, AR 72701

Phone: (479) 521-9195

THE SCHOOL OF INTEGRATIVE NUTRITION

New York City

www.integrativenutrition.com

A holistic nutrition school integrating all different dietary theories, from the ancient traditions of ayurveda, macrobiotics and Chinese medicine to the most current concepts like raw foods, Atkins diet, blood type diets, the Zone and the USDA Healthy Eating Pyramid.

MIDWEST

∘ ∘ ∘

BOB CARR

Director: East West Center of Cleveland (1984–present)

Macrobiotic Teacher/Counselor

Taught Oriental Medicine & Shiatsu at Ohio College of Massotherapy 1995

Author of *The Energy of Food*, 1992

Taught at Kushi Institute Northern Europe 1990-91

Director of the Macrobiotic Center of Munich (Germany) 1989

Editor of MacroNewsLetter (e-mail newsletter)

Founded Cleveland Tofu Co. 1980

2471 Derbyshire Rd.

Cleveland Heights, OH 44106

Phone: (216) 321-0139

Email: RNCJR@apk.net

JANET VITT, R.N., B.S.N.

Macrobiotic Counselor/Cook/Teacher/Stage IV Lung Cancer Survivor

Phone: (330) 467-6739

NATURAL RESEARCH AND HEALING ARTS

Stefan Brink Ac.T.

1120 N. Washington

Royal Oak, MI 48067

Natural Research and Healing Arts offers Macrobiotic Counseling, Traditional Chinese Medicine including Acupuncture, Tui Na, Chinese Herbs, some Western Herbs and Homeopathy, Colon Hydrotherapy, Cranial Sacral Therapy, Rolf Structural Integration, and has a medical intuitive on staff.

GABRIELLE F. KUSHI

Macrobiotic Level IV Certified Practitioner

Consulting, in person, over the phone or vial e-mail

Chef services, cooking instruction

Minneapolis - St. Paul, MN

Phone: (612) 834-1476

www.kushiskitchen.com

FRANCOIS ROLAND

Macrobiotic counselor, cook/teacher

Email: macrocenter@yahoo.com

Phone: (216) 371-3222

JOHN KOZINSKI, MEA

Senior Macrobiotic Counselor

Chicago, IL

30 years counseling seriously ill and healthy lifestyle seekers using modern approaches including diet/complementary modalities.

Phone: (413) 623-5925

www.macrobiotic.com

WEST

o o o

DAVID BRISCOE

David Briscoe has been teaching and counseling macrobiotics for over 30 years. He is regularly invited to be a guest faculty member at events of the Kushi Institute. The George Ohsawa Macrobiotic Foundation, and the Health Classics. David has presented macrobiotic programs at hospitals, cancer centers, and other health organizations. He currently runs Macrobiotics America in California.

Macrobiotics America
P.O. Box 1874
Oroville, CA 95965
www.macroamerica.com
Phone: (530) 532-1918

MEREDITH MCCARTY

San Francisco, CA

Meredith McCarty, DC, NE, is a holistic nutritionist (Diet Counselor and Nutrition Educator) and is founder of www.healingcuisine.com. She has authored three macrobiotic cookbooks and produced a video. Formerly the associate editor of Natural Health magazine, Meredith co-directed a macrobiotic center in northern California for 19 years, during which time she catered weekly dinner parties and annual residential seminars for up to 150 people. She has consulted, taught and lectured internationally since 1977. Meredith currently resides in the San Francisco Bay Area.

Healing Cuisine Macrobiotic consultations (in person or by phone), cooking classes, lectures, cookbooks, monthly e-newsletter
P.O. Box 2605
Mill Valley, CA 94942
Phone: (415) 381-1735
www.healingcuisine.com

GEORGE OSHAWA MACROBIOTICS FOUNDATION

Carl & Julia Ferre

P.O. Box 3998

Chico, CA 95927-3998

Phone: (530) 566-9765

       (800) 232-2372

www.gomf.macrobiotic.net

Publishes books and Macrobiotic Today magazine, conduct the Annual French Meadows camps and providedd contacts to macrobiotics persons throughout the world. Carl Ferre is the author of *The Pocket Guide to Macrobiotics* and the compiler of Essential Oshawa. Julia Ferre is the author of *The Basics of Macrobiotic Cooking*.

FRED PULVER

Carbondale, CO

Phone: (970) 963-0229

Email: fred@macrobiotic.org

Fred Pulver, of Carbondale, Colorado, is a Macrobiotic Counselor, writer and educator. He studied and worked with Michio Kushi, Herman Aihara, and Noburo Muramoto. Fred assisted the compilation of GOMF publications, translated articles from French, and wrote for and edited Macrobiotics Today magazine, in San Francisco and Oroville, CA in the 1970's. He now maintains an active website at www.macrobiotic.org.

YUKA FUKADA

Macrobiotic counseling, cooking, and classes.

Eugene, Oregon

Phone: 541-342-3994

Email: ecofamily@nifty.com

www.ecofamily.info

INTERNATIONAL

o o o

JANET SCOTT

Cape Town, South Africa

Macrobiotic guidance, workshops and cooking classes

Email: janetscott@discoverymail.co.za

JAMIE TREVENA

Great Britain

Website Host – The Macrobiotic Guide

www.macrobiotics.co.uk

THE KUSHI INSTITUTE OF EUROPE

Weteringschans 65

1017 RX Amsterdam, RX

Phone: +31 (0) 20 625 75 13

Fax: +31 (0) 20 622 73 20

Email: kushi@macrobiotics.nl

SHELDIN AND GUNAT RICE

Israel

www.thericehouse.com: Offers insights into macrobiotics, numerology, nine star ki, shiatsu and palmistry. Also offers a variety of on site programs including cooking classes, seminars, theory classes and spa days.

LIFE COACHES

○ ○ ○

SALLY McCUE

Professional Life Coach for Individuals and Groups

P.O. Box 864

York Harbor, Maine 03911

Email: GrowthWork@aol.com

www.growthwork.net

JOAN BORGATTI

Author, Motivational Speaker and Life Coach

212 Worcester Street

Wellesley Hills, MA 02481

www.joanborgatti.com

DR. MARTHA BECK

Author and Life Coach

Email: martha@marthabeck.com

www.marthabeck.com

JADE WOOD

North Star Certified Life Coach

Phone: (510) 520-2345

Email: jadetwood@aol.com

• • •

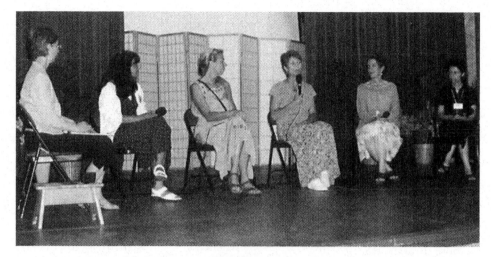

AFTERWORD

Fall 2005

I feel fortunate to be alive and well today. Because of macrobiotics, I was able to see my son graduate from high school and go on to college and to celebrate my daughter's sixteenth birthday—another milestone I feared I would never see. And, I have a future with my husband, Tom, as we continue our life's purpose of helping others in their journey towards health.

This summer I attended the Kushi Institute Summer Conference, where I spoke on a panel of breast cancer survivors who were healed through macrobiotics. Among the women on the panel was Bonnie Kramer, who had inspired me at the first Kushi Institute conference. It was a wonderful confirmation in how far I had come in my healing—from an ill spectator to a healthy woman advocating the macrobiotic way of life for others.

In the fall, Tom and I attended a life-changing workshop at the Omega Institute in New York. The workshop called, "Getting the Love You Want", was taught by Harville Hendrix and Helen LeKelly Hunt. We were taught Imago dialogue and learned the valuable processes to work through strong emotions to a place of clarity, understanding, and connection. This was the best marriage therapy we have ever experienced, and we are committed to this process.

Now that my leg has healed, I will be getting a new artificial leg. My new goal is to be extremely mobile and to dance up a storm!

Look out, Broadway!

o o o

INDEX

∘ ∘ ∘

CPSIA information can be obtained at www.ICGtesting.com
Printed in the USA
BVOW09s1053060816

458100BV00002B/10/P